Flowers
& fables

Flowers
& *fables*
A Welsh Herbal

Jocelyne Lawton

seren

Seren is the book imprint of
Poetry Wales Press Ltd
57 Nolton Street, Bridgend, CF31 3AE,
www.seren-books.com

ISBN 1-85411-407-7

A CIP record for this title is available from
the British Library.

The publisher works with the financial assistance of the
Welsh Books Council.

Printed in Perpetua by Gwasg Gomer

Flowers and Fables is a work of reference and entertainment. Flowers, herbs and fungi can be dangerous if misused and the author and publisher can bear no responsibility for the medical claims of folklore and history described in this book. If the healing powers of plants are of interest to you, please
consult a qualified specialist in herbal remedies.

Excellent herbs had our fathers of old —
Excellent herbs to ease their pain —
Alexanders and Marigold,
Eyebright, Orris and Elecampane —
Basil, Rocket, Valerian, Rue,
(Almost singing themselves they run)
Vervain, Dittany, Call-me-to-you —
Cowslip, Melilot, Rose of the Sun.
Anything green that grew out of the mould
Was an excellent herb to our fathers of old.

Wonderful tales had our fathers of old,
Wonderful tales of the herbs and the stars —
The Sun was Lord of the Marigold,
Basil and Rocket belonged to Mars.
Pat as a sum in division it goes —
(Every herb had a planet bespoke) —
Who but Venus should govern the Rose?
Who but Jupiter own the Oak?
Simply and gravely the facts are told
In the wonderful books of our fathers of old.

From 'Our fathers of old', *Rewards and Fairies,* Rudyard Kipling

I wish to dedicate this book to my husband and children, without whose help, encouragement and occasional threats it would not have been finished. I would also like to mention a venerable ginger cat, who used to get very bored if I spent too long taking the photographs and who often sat on the keyboard, generating some very peculiar typescript.

Introduction

For many centuries, and perhaps for all of history, flowers have been important to the human race. They are attractive and colourful, some are spectacular, many are sweet scented. It was perhaps natural in the days before systematic medicine, or indeed any medicine at all, that ailing people should turn to flowers for relief. It is likely that in primitive societies these blooms were regarded as gifts of the gods and, to people who were wise enough to recognise them, would have had many valuable properties. This was undoubtedly the case, but the interaction of medical properties with religious significance led to much confusion and the rise of folklore and superstitions. By the fifteenth century the properties of flowers were beginning to be methodically recorded in 'herbals' of which many survive, perhaps the best known being that of Nicholas Culpeper, *The Complete Herbal*, published in 1649. These deal primarily with the medical properties of herbs. (In this context, a 'herb' simply means a plant which does not have a woody stem.) The superstitions and folklore were largely handed down by word of mouth, and varied widely from region to region.

Country people were very superstitious. Obviously they were very much afraid of thunder, especially lightning which was a threat to their thatched homes, hay ricks or crops, so they used to hang ox-eye daisies around the doors of their houses, on the roof and the haylofts to give them protection. Farmers believed strongly in the powerful mysticism of flowers – they would even rub their cows' udders with buttercups to give them a better yield. Flowers were also used for divination by young girls seeking husbands, for example sowing butterbur seeds on a Friday evening was said to reveal a vision of your future husband mowing a meadow. In general, flowers were very important to country people not only for medicine but for divination, poison (you could do away with your neighbour) or for predicting the weather. Flowers would do it all. These and many other stories I have included in this book.

While *Flowers and Fables* should enable you to recognise many of the more common wild flowers, it also contains stories from folklore and early medical recipes and remedies belonging to each plant. In addition close-up photographs of the flowers show them in considerable detail including aspects not normally visible to the naked eye.

I have also given explanations of the naming histories of each plant, some of which can be traced back to the Ancient Greeks. Since folk legends are transmitted by word of mouth, they inevitably become changed over the centuries, and my versions may differ from the ones you know. Both the writing and photography were undertaken in Wales, and I have also given, where applicable, the names of each flower in Welsh as well as in English. Details of Welsh folklore are included too.

The third name given for each flower is the scientific name. The system for naming all organisms was laid down by Carolus Linnaeus in 1735. Linnaeus was a Swedish botanist who devised binomial nomenclature, a double name for each species, for example *Primula vulgaris*, the common primrose. The first name is the *generic name*, which defines the genus or group to which the plant belongs. The second name is the *specific name* which refers to the species, or the particular type of plant. Scientific names are standardised and internationally recognised. The names are popularly supposed to be of Latin origin, but are as frequently derived from Greek and are normally descriptive of the plant or may refer to some aspect of the folklore. In *Primula vulgaris* for instance *Primula* is Latin for 'little first one' (of the spring) and *vulgaris* simply means 'common'. The bluebell (*Endymion nonscriptus*) is named after Endymion, a character of Greek legend.

As stated, flowers were an essential ingredient in early medicine. Welsh medicine is thought to date from the beginning of the thirteenth century. Rhys Gryg (known as Rhys the Hoarse), was a son of Rhys ap Gruffydd. He was a Prince of south Wales, a good soldier and was much involved with the feuds of the time. He had a physician who was called Rhiwallon, who was assisted by his three sons, Cadwgan, Gruffydd and Einion. They lived in the village of Myddfai in Carmarthenshire and were known as The Physicians of Myddfai.

With the support and protection of Rhys Gryg, the physicians made and wrote down a large collection of medical recipes, involving the use of herbs. Many of these herbal remedies can be traced back to the time of Hywel Dda, but it was the Myddfai Physicians who collected and recorded them, thus making the knowledge available to us today.

Many legends surround the Physicians of Myddfai, one of the best known is 'The Lady of the Lake'. This tells the story of a young man who used to take his cattle to graze beside and drink from a small lake called Llyn-y-Fan-Fach on the north west side of the Carmarthenshire Fans in the Black Mountains. One day, while the young man was walking beside the shores of the lake, he saw to his intense surprise the most beautiful girl he had ever seen. She appeared to be sitting on the surface of the water. Not surprisingly he fell helplessly in love with her, and offered her the coarse barley bread and cheese that he had with him. This she refused. Twice more he offered her some of his bread, until it was finally to her liking. After some persuasion she accepted his offer of marriage promising that they would live together in harmony, unless he struck her three times without any reason. After the third blow, she would leave him forever and return to her father beneath the waters of the lake. So the young couple were married and lived at a farm called Esgair Llaethdy near the village of Myddfai. They were very happy together and they had three handsome and clever sons.

Over a period of years, while their sons grew up, he struck his wife three times without cause, and she held her destiny fulfilled, left him and returned to Llyn-y-Fan-Fach with all the livestock she had brought as a dowry. On reaching the lake she disappeared beneath the water without trace.

What became of the distracted and ruined husband is not known, but the three boys used to walk along the shore of the lake often, hoping they might see their mother. During one of these walks, the mother appeared to her eldest son, Rhiwallon, at the 'Llidiad y Meddygon', the 'Physicians' gate'. She told him he would be a great physician and a benefactor of mankind by relieving them of pain and misery through the healing of all diseases. She then gave him a bag full of prescriptions with instructions on how to make them. She appeared on several more occasions to her sons, showing them the various plants and teaching them about their medicinal properties. The knowledge that she passed on to her sons, together with their own unrivalled skill, made them into the legendary Physicians of Myddfai, the founders of Welsh medicine.

It is important to remember the part that folklore and magic played in rural communities. Not all healing was based on reason and observation. Every village would have had its 'wise man' or 'wise woman' who, for a consideration, would dispense wisdom or remedies, frequently based on flowers, for almost any affliction, whether of body or soul, human or animal.

Another example of this in Wales was the Wise Men of Llangurig. Two well known members of the 'wise men' were Evan Griffiths from Pant-y-Benni, Llangurig, and Edward Davies, of Y Fagwyr Fawr, Ponterwyd. They taught themselves the arts of healing from books and were both well respected for their talent at curing animals. So much so in fact that people from north and mid Wales actually believed them capable of supernatural powers to cure and protect livestock. In return for payment the wise man would write, in illegible handwriting, a charm on a piece of paper in a mixture of Welsh, English and Latin. This included a prayer for bewitched animals or a blessing for protection against witchcraft, some magic incantations and, finally, various signs of the zodiac. This charm was then sealed inside a small bottle called 'potel y dyn hysbys' (the knowing one's bottle). This was given to the farmer, who would hide it in the building where the animals were kept, with the instruction that the cork should never be removed.

Well, the Wise Men of Llangurig are long gone, and the Physicians of Myddfai are no more. In their place we have the National Health Service which, whatever its virtues, is perhaps less colourful. No longer do we have to chew willow bark to cure a headache or daisy leaves to cure mouth ulcers, although many plant-derived remedies are still with us today in modified forms. Where superstitions are concerned, children will still blow dandelion clocks to tell the time, but I think few young girls will use butterbur or ragged robin to divine the names of their future sweethearts.

Should you wish to try this as an alternative to a dating agency, please feel free to do so, but please remember some of these plants used incautiously may prove lethal. You have been warned! I will accept no responsibility whatsoever for any results obtained by the use of any of the methods used in this book, but I hope the stories here presented will provide some entertainment on a country walk.

Bee Orchid
Tegeirian y Gwenyn
Ophrys apifera

Description

Of all the British orchids the bee orchid is perhaps the best known and certainly the most easily recognised. Up to 40cm tall, the single fleshy stem carries two or three complex flowers. The slender leaves grow at intervals on the stem. Like many other flowers they need the services of insects to pollinate them, and have gone to remarkable lengths to recruit these unwitting helpers. The flower bears a surprising resemblance to the rear of a bumble bee that is apparently visiting it to obtain nectar. This may prove attractive to other bees, which then become inflamed with passion and attempt to mate with it. This will be beneficial to the flower, since the bee will become covered with pollen, which it will then transfer to the other flowers and cross pollinate them. It will not, however, benefit the bee, which will have a frustrating day.

Habitat

Bee orchids are quite often found growing in groups, and where one is found it is likely others will be nearby. They like growing on calcareous grassland, open oak and pine woods, on banks and in copses, especially on chalky or clay-like soils. These plants are protected by law.

Naming History

This flower used to be called the 'humble-bee orchis', since it mimics the bumble bee and not the honey bee. The name 'humble' or 'bumble' bee comes from the familiar droning or humming sound that this very large insect makes in flight. This is signified by some of the other local names for this flower, including 'humble-bee flower' from Kent, 'honey-flower' from Surrey and from Somerset 'dumble dor', which is an old country name for a bumble bee.

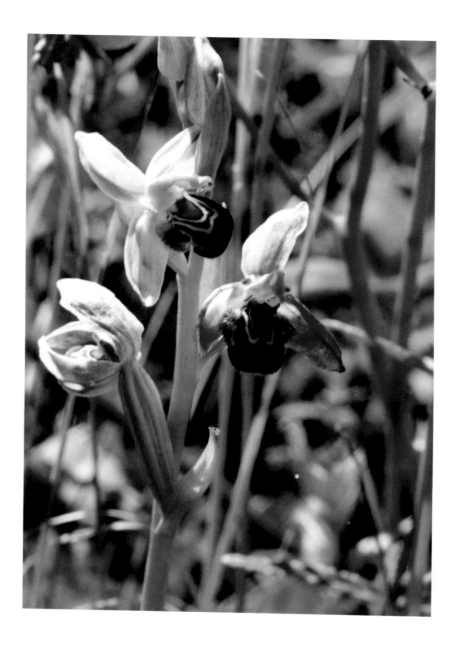

Bee Orchid

Bird's-foot Trefoil
Basged Bysgota, Pys y Ceirw
Lotus corniculatus

Description

Bird's-foot trefoil is a low-creeping, downy perennial that entwines itself into long grass. The leaves have five leaflets, the lowest pair being bent back so that the leaves appear trefoil. The flowers bloom through from May to September. They are yellow, pea-shaped and often tinged with orange or red. After the flowers die back, the fruiting pods appear, usually between four and six to a head.

Habitat

On a hot summer's day in a meadow, amid the buzzing of grasshoppers, the eye may be drawn to small yellow flowers between the grass stems. This is the favoured habitat of bird's-foot trefoil.

Naming History

This plant gains its name from the arrangement of its fruiting pods which has the appearance of a bird's foot, and the term 'trefoil' comes from the three-lobed leaves. The definition of the generic name *Lotus* is not known, except that the name probably came from the classical Greek *lotos*, and was applied to an extensive variety of plants. However the specific name *corniculatus*, meaning 'possessing small horns' also relates to the shape of the fruiting pods.

Some other country names include 'bird's claws', 'bird's eye' and 'bird's foot' from Devon; 'boots-and-shoes' from Somerset; 'boxing gloves', 'bread-and-cheese' and 'bunny rabbit's ears' from Sussex and 'butter-and-eggs' from Somerset.

Folklore

Bird's-foot trefoil is a little plant that has been endowed with over seventy country names. Some of these names refer to the flowers, and some to the seed pods. As stated, these pods can have an uncanny resemblance to birds' or animals' claws and even the claws of a hag, or other images that were considered evil, such as the claws of the crow, the evil cat and even the fingers of the Devil. It was therefore considered that this plant needed converting and it was made into a plant of God and the Virgin. In some rural counties in England, bird's-foot trefoil is also known as 'Tom Thumb', 'hop-o-my-thumb' and 'Jack-jump-about'. Originally Tom Thumb was a supernaturally powerful, pixie-like figure, considered capable of taking drastic magical revenge if offended. This association rendered the flower unlucky to pick, but not to everyone. In the South of Ireland children gathered the plant to take to school with them, believing that possessing it would protect them from punishment. It was said that they would travel miles to find it.

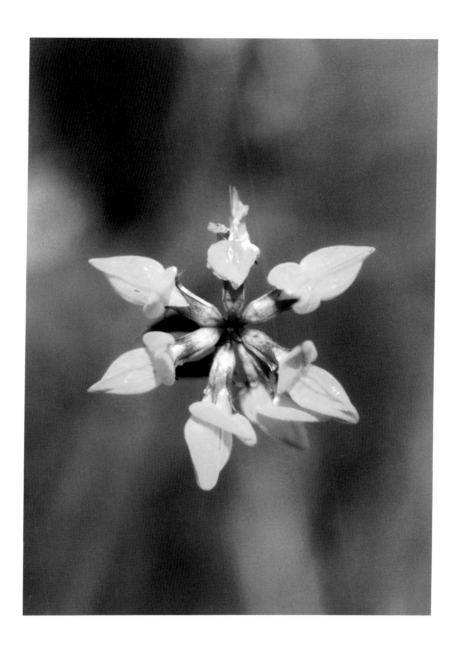

Bird's-Foot Trefoil

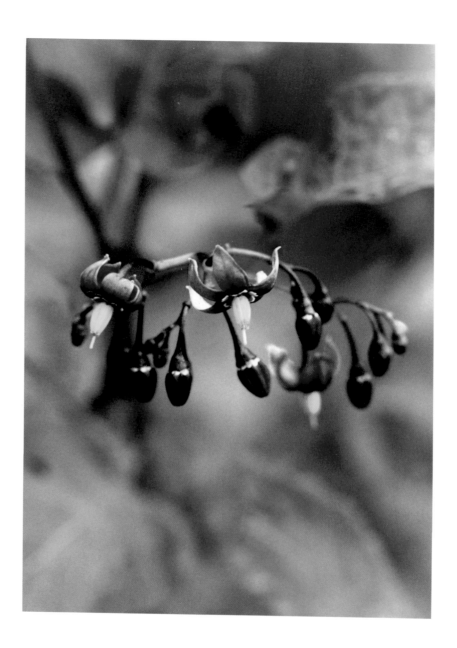

Bittersweet (Woody Nightshade)

Bittersweet (Woody Nightshade)
Mochlys, Codwarth Caled
Solanum dulcamara

Description

This climbing perennial has oval pointed leaves, often with two lobes at the base. It can be easily recognised in the hedgerows by its small but distinctive flowers which appear between July and October. These grow in loose clusters, the petals are a vibrant purple and the yellow anthers grow in a characteristic spike. After the flowers have served their purpose, they swell to become green, poisonous berries, later flushing red.

Habitat

Bittersweet possesses tendrils and it can entwine itself into hedges, which it uses for its support. It is a common plant and is often found growing in woods, scrub, waste areas and damp places.

Naming History

The specific name *dulcamara* (bittersweet) describes the berries' first bitter then sweet taste (obviously for health and safety reasons you should not try this yourself). The name 'woody nightshade' indicates that the plant is a woody perennial, unlike its close and herbaceous relative, the perennial black nightshade. The name 'nightshade' may have derived from an early medical name '*solatrum*' which was commonly mistaken for '*solem atrum*' meaning 'shade as of night' or 'black sun'. Pliny gave the generic name *Solanum* which came from the Latin *solamen*, 'solace' or *solor* meaning comfort because of the narcotic effects of some species. Perhaps the most likely is that the name came from the Latin *sol*, 'sun' because of the characteristic shape of the flowers although latterly the name might have come from the Latin *sus*, since the plant could be used to treat pigs for some disorders. William Turner gave it the name of bittersweet, when he wrote his *Herbal* in 1568. Other names include 'felonwood' and 'felonwort', the former being a corruption of the latter which means 'the felon's plant'.

Folklore

Plants which happen to produce red berries were often regarded as having magical properties, and bittersweet was no exception. It was considered to be a charm against witchcraft and in Lincolnshire collars of bittersweet were hung around 'overlooked' pigs to protect them. (I have not found out exactly what this means, but it seems possible that a runt, a piglet ignored by its mother, might merit this description.) In other country areas garlands of holly and bittersweet were hung around the necks of 'hagridden' horses, and similarly in Germany garlands were hung round the necks of cattle to protect them from evil. It could be used for people as well. In Norfolk, necklaces were made from dried nightshade berries and placed around the necks of babies to prevent them from having convulsions. Culpeper mentioned it as an excellent remedy to "remove Witchcraft from men and beasts".

Other uses including medicinal

Bittersweet had many uses and it was introduced into medicine by German physicians in the sixteenth century. You could use the stalks to treat rheumatism and skin diseases and as a purgative. Vertigo or dizziness could be relieved by tying a bit of the plant around the neck (assuming that you had some to hand) and, should you be troubled with whitlows (an abscess near a fingernail or toenail), bruising the berries and applying them to the troubled area would eliminate the problem. A Cotswold remedy for chilblains was to rub in the berries of bittersweet. Indeed this remedy was so well regarded that the berries were stored in bottles for the forthcoming winter.

Black Knapweed
Pengaled
Centaurea nigra

Description

This common, medium to tall perennial is often mistaken for a thistle. The flowers, which appear during the summer months of June to September, are composed of a cluster of purple florets emerging from dark brown to black, sepal-like bracts. Unlike the thistle, however, this plant is not spiny.

Habitat

Black knapweed likes flowering in dry, grassy areas. It is a common sight in the summer, growing in meadows and along the roadsides.

Naming History

As described, the sepal-like bracts at the base of the flowers are very dark giving rise to the specific name of *nigra* meaning 'black'. The common name 'knapweed' is corrupted from the word 'knop', or 'knopweed', because of the toughness of the plant and the shape of the flower buds, 'knop' being corrupted from 'knob'. They were also known as 'hardheads' because of this, and possibly also because of the bud's resemblance to a loggerhead, an iron ball on a long handle, used to heat pitch for caulking ships' seams.

The generic name *Centaurea* is after the Centaur Chiron who, in Greek mythology, used a similar plant to heal the wounds he received on his foot from a poisoned arrow which had been soaked in the blood of the Hydra. After this Chiron taught Achilles and other heroes the arts of medicine, music and hunting. As a reward, the god Zeus placed him in heaven among the stars as Sagittarius.

Folklore

Some country names such as 'bachelor's buttons', from Ireland and 'Bobby's buttons', from Somerset, indicate that black knapweed was sometimes used for divination. Young girls would pick the buds and place them inside their blouses. After a while they took them out to see if the buds had opened with the help of the warmth of their bodies. If any had, this was thought to indicate that love had been requited.

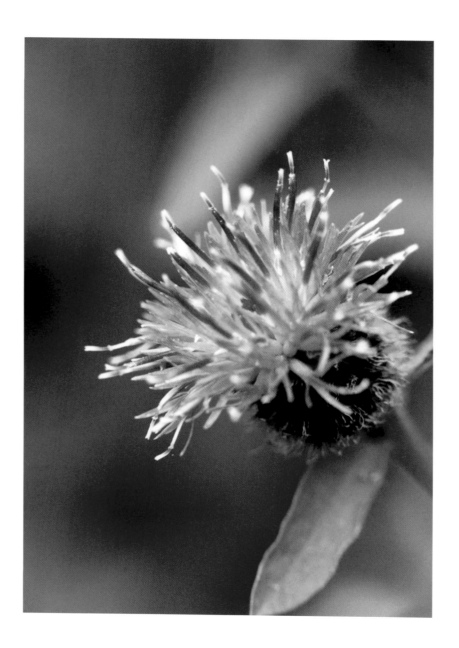

Black Knapweed

Some other charming names are 'chimneysweep' and 'chimneysweep's brushes' from Somerset, and 'clobweed' from Gloucestershire.

Other uses including medicinal

Black knapweed is a popular herb with modern herbalists. It is a useful astringent and is used in the treatment of piles. A decoction of the herb can be used as a gargle, giving relief to sore throats.

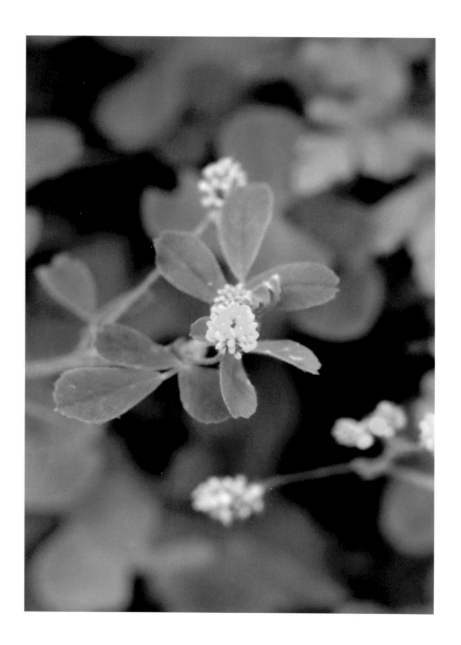

Black Medick

Black Medick
Maglys
Medicago lupulina

Description

This common, downy, low-creeping annual can be easily recognised by its trefoil-shaped leaves and small round yellow flowers, so small, in fact, that it is often overlooked. The stems may be up to 40cm long, with the flowers growing in clusters at the tips. The individual flowers are only about three millimetres across.

Habitat

Black medick can be found flowering throughout the summer from April to October. It favours bare and grassy places, and can often be found growing on or beside footpaths and road verges.

Naming History

The ripe seed pods are black and curved, giving the plant its name of black medick, and some of its attractive local names, such as 'black nonesuch' from Buckinghamshire, 'fingers-and-thumbs' from Somerset and 'lamb's toes' from Northumberland, emphasise this. The specific name *lupulina* means 'hop-like', and was given because of the flower's (albeit fancied) resemblance to hops (*Humulus lupulus*).

Folklore

It is believed that Dioscorides, a Greek physician from Anazarbus in Cilicia, gave the plant its generic name of *medike*. The name 'medick' has nothing to do with medicinal qualities, but actually means the Medean herb or herb of the Medes. The Medes were a fifth century BC people who appear in the biblical story of the prophet Daniel. During the feast given by the Babylonian king Belshazzar, the mysterious writing which appeared on the wall warned about the imminent invasion of Babylon by the Medes and the Persians. Dioscorides was also the author of *De Materia Medica*, which was used as a herbal reference for many years. In his herbal he describes the Medean herb as being similar to the crop lucerne, which was used as cattle fodder in those times.

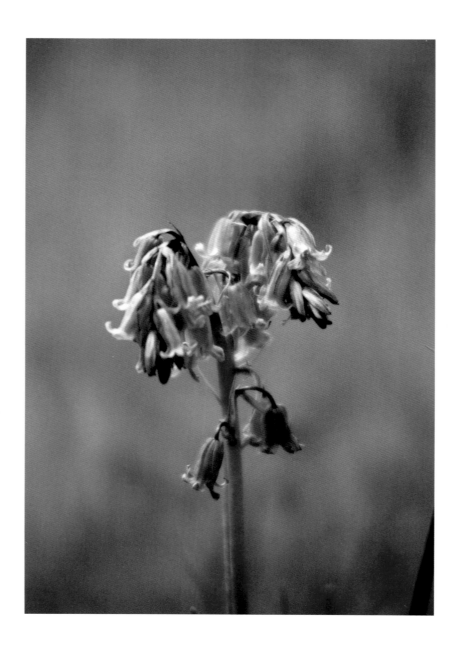

Bluebell

Bluebell
Clychau'r Gôg
Endymion non-scriptus

Description

These beautiful, well known flowers cover the woods of Britain in springtime with a brilliant blue carpet. The straight fleshy leaves, growing in tufts, surround a flower spike of up to twenty hanging bells, varying in colour from deep violet almost to white. Few other flowers grow in the woods at this time, and the bluebells are spectacularly dominant. You may observe some bluebells which are slightly larger than normal and which have flowers on both sides of the stem. These are Spanish bluebells, an introduced species which is rapidly spreading and, in places, taking over. The native bluebell has flowers on one side of the stem only.

Habitat

The majority of lowland woods in Britain are deciduous, comprising a variety of trees. The bluebell flowers before most leaves emerge, in the brief period when sunlight reaches the woodland floor and, when the shade increases towards the end of spring, the flowers die back to leave the bulbous seedheads.

Naming history

The common name 'bluebell' is self-explanatory, but the plant has had other identities in the past. The plant was originally associated with the hyacinth family, a name which derives from the legendary Greek youth Hyakinthos, son of a Spartan prince. The human youth was befriended by Apollo, the Greek god of music and healing, who showed him many favours. This created jealousy in the west wind, also a special friend of Apollo. One day, as Apollo was teaching Hyakinthos to throw the discus, the west wind seized his opportunity and blew the discus back into Hyakinthos' face, injuring him severely, and where his blood fell, the first hyacinth flower sprang. The bluebell has a resemblance to the hyacinth, but was later reclassified into a separate family. Greek legend is also the origin of the generic name *Endymion*, after the young Greek shepherd of that name, with whom the moon goddess Selene fell in love as he slept on the hillside.

The specific name *non-scriptus* means 'unmarked' and is a reference to the plain blue petals, in contrast to the streaks or lines on the petals of the hyacinth.

The Welsh name *clychau'r gôg* translates as 'cuckoo bells' since the flowers are seen at about the same time the cuckoo is heard.

Bramble
Miaren
Rubus fruticosus

Description

The well known and heavily armed bramble is found in all parts of Britain. Abundant long, strong, sprawling stems well provided with stout spines support dull green, oval, slightly toothed leaves which may persist through most of the year, except where winter is particularly severe.

The flowers of the bramble appear in Maytime, and are white, tinged with pale pink. They are usually about 20-30mm across, with a corolla of yellow anthers in the centre. In the autumn, the flowers develop into the familiar fruit that we call the blackberry. The unripe fruit is red, ripening to black, providing food for hungry birds as well as for us, although in many parts of England it is said to be unlucky to pick blackberries after Michaelmas, for then the devil is said to have spat on them.

Habitat

This scrambling, thorny shrub grows in woods, scrub, open and waste ground, in addition to being an extremely unwelcome visitor in many gardens. It can be found entwined into hedgerows and along roadsides, as well as growing out in the open in meadows. In fact bramble grows prolifically, up to three inches a day in good conditions, and where a shoot touches the ground it will frequently root itself. The stems are not really self-supporting, and this, combined with the speed of growth, produces an intricate mass of scrub which effectively chokes out other plants. The bramble is not particular about soil conditions and will grow enthusiastically in almost any ground.

Naming History

The name 'bramble' is used throughout England, Scotland and Ireland, although it varies according to the dialect e.g. 'brimmel', 'brummel' and 'bummel', although some counties will have their own local names, notably 'lady's garters' from Somerset and 'country lawyers' from Worcestershire. Names for the fruit include 'blaggs' or 'bleggs' in Yorkshire and in Cumberland 'doctor's medicine'.

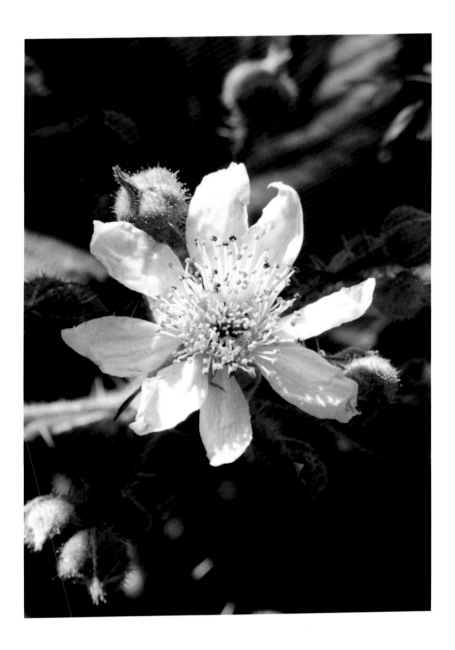

Bramble

Folklore

In the days before more precise medicine, Cornish folk believed that many diseases would be cured if the sufferer walked under an arch of bramble that was rooted at both ends. Bramble will put out suckers and, where a shoot touches the ground, it will frequently root itself forming a natural arch. This led to a Welsh belief that children who were suffering from rickets, or who were slow to walk, should crawl or creep under a bramble bush three times a week hopefully to cure their condition. Until as late as 1978 a Staffordshire cure for whooping cough was to find a similar arch on a bramble bush, and pass the child through it and over it nine times on three mornings a week before sunrise chanting:

> Under the briar, and over the briar,
> I wish to leave the chin cough here.

In County Kerry in Ireland, they had quite a different belief. Until 1947 they believed that if a person walked under a bramble bush that had both ends in the ground, and at the same time gave themselves up to the Devil, they should win themselves good luck in card playing!

As stated, the speedy growth of the bramble and the facility of rooting the ends of the stems forms the thick, tangled scrub we are all familiar with. The impenetrability of these tangles led to an English custom whereby graves in churchyards would be planted round with brambles to restrain the dead from walking.

Less prosaically, Scottish Highlanders would twine together wreaths of bramble, rowan and ivy to hang over their doorways as a protection from witches and evil spirits, since it was said that Jesus Christ had driven out the money lenders from the temple with a switch made from bramble, and used the same to encourage the donkey on his way into Jerusalem. The bramble was thus hallowed by association and it was therefore believed that witches and evil spirits would fear to pass it.

Wandering sheep would frequently get caught in brambles leaving strands of wool on the thorns and this free supply would be gratefully received by country housewives for spinning to make clothes for the family. This leads to the very attractive story about the bat, the cormorant and the bramble. It was said that the cormorant was once a wool merchant. He decided to go shares with the bat and the bramble in a boat, to export his wool abroad. There was a terrible storm and the boat was wrecked on some rocks. So now the cormorant is always diving after his lost cargo, the bat owes money and hides from its creditors till dark, and the bramble makes up its losses by stealing wool from the sheep.

It has always been considered unlucky to pick and eat blackberries after Michaelmas Day, 11th October. According to legend the Devil fell into a bramble bush when he was cast out of heaven, and spat on the blackberries in annoyance at his lost dignity. He returned to the bush again on St Simon's day, 28th October, and trod an irate path around the bush, to make sure that no more blackberries would appear after that date. A Worcestershire correspondent in the 1972 September issue of *Country Life*, wrote that the disfigurement of the leaves caused by leaf miner grubs was known as 'devil's marks'. In some parts of England, it is said that witches ruined the blackberries, whilst in Ireland the Bogey Pooka (Puka or Phooka) is said to have ruined them. But a period of fine weather at the end of September, early October when the blackberries were ripening was known as a 'blackberry summer'.

Other uses including medicinal

The Scottish Highlanders used the roots to make an orange dye, and the leaves were placed on burns and used to reduce swellings, a remedy that was still used by the sixteenth-century herbalists. Perhaps an extension of this was the tradition whereby bramble leaves were used with a charm to cure scalds. Nine leaves soaked in spring water would be applied to the injury and the following charm recited:

> There came three angels from the East.
> One brought fire, and two brought frost.
> Out fire, in frost!
> In the name of Father, Son and Holy Ghost.

Broom
Banadl
Sarothamnus scoparius

Description

This tall deciduous shrub can be easily recognised by its bright yellow, leguminous or pea-like flowers, which appear in late spring from April to June. The upright stems, which are ridged and slightly waxy, give rise to short side branches bearing short light green leaves. Unlike the rather similar gorse, the broom has no spines.

In late summer the flowers give rise to small dry black pods containing the seeds. On hot summer days the sun will dry the pods to the point where they will split with an audible cracking sound, and the two halves, swiftly curling back on themselves, will fling the seeds to a surprising distance. Indeed, on a suitable day, a bush of broom will emit a continuous crackling sound as the seeds are dispersed.

Habitat

Broom is a very common shrub, and is widespread in Britain and western Europe. It likes to grow on dry acid soils, but can occasionally be seen on chalk and limestone. It can usually be found growing on heaths and in open woodland.

Naming History

The name 'broom' simply refers to the early use of the twigs for sweeping. It is not clear however, whether the word was originally applied to the shrub or to the implement. As can be readily imagined the twigs of broom would sweep well, but would also wear out fairly quickly (especially on the earthen floors popular in mediaeval times) and, becoming less effective, would require replacement. Hence the proverb 'a new broom sweeps clean'.

This is further illustrated by the generic name *Sarothamnus*, *saron* from the Greek meaning 'besom', an old name for broom, and *thamnos* meaning 'shrub'. In addition the specific name *scoparius* also means 'brush' or 'broom-like'. When Welsh authors and people are describing something yellow it is a common phrase for them to say it is 'felyn fel blodau'r banadl' or 'yellow like broom flowers'.

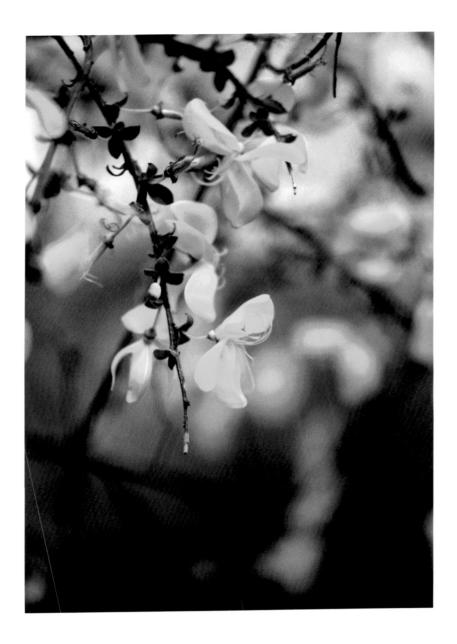

Broom

Folklore

Country people were very superstitious, and broom was considered to have some very sinister qualities. One was that it was thought unlucky to sweep the house with twigs which still had blossom on them. This is signified by an old Sussex rhyme which says:

> If you sweep the house with blossomed broom in May,
> You'll sweep the head of the house away.

Or a similar rhyme from Reading, which has an even worse association;

> If you bring broom into the house in May
> It will sweep the family away.

It could also act as a domestic oracle. Another rhyme tells about an over-loquacious wife consulting the spirit of the broom:

> Tell me, being in the broom,
> Teach me what to do
> That my husband
> Love me true?
>
> When your tongue is still
> You'll have your will.

However despite its associations, and because of its profusion of bright yellow flowers, a bundle of green broom tied with ribbons often appeared at country weddings as a symbol of good luck and plenty. It was also hung in houses as a Whitsuntide decoration, probably because of the many yellow and orange flowers resembling the tongues of fire descending onto the disciples, enabling them to converse in many languages.

Other uses including medicinal

England was ruled by the Plantagenets for almost two hundred and fifty years, and it was the Plantagenet kings who fought in the Hundred Years War against the French. The name Plantagenet was a nickname for Geoffrey of Anjou, the founder of the dynasty. He and his men always wore a sprig of broom into battle, so that they could be recognised by their own side. However the name does not appear to have been adopted by the royal family until the mid 1400s, so some historians prefer to refer to Henry II and his sons as Angevins.

Towards the end of the seventeenth century, broom buds were considered a rare delicacy. They were pickled in vinegar and served at the coronation feast of James II as an hors d'oeuvre. They were also used to add the bitter flavour in beer, before the introduction of hops.

As a medicinal plant, broom was said to be good for cleansing the kidneys and bladder, as a general diuretic and for easing joint pains.

Butterbur
Dail Tryfan
Petasites hybridus

Description

The flowers appear before the leaves during the spring months of March to May. They are strange looking blooms, a short thick flower spike bearing whorls of small white flowers in the centre. The heart-shaped leaves are very large and can be up to one metre across. Country people used to use these leaves as umbrellas, following the recommendation of Gerard who said that "the leaf is of such a widenesse as that of itselfe it is bigge and large enough to keepe a man's head from raine and from the heate of the sun". Unfortunately, in practice, the rain just runs down the leaf's guttering and soaks you anyway.

Habitat

These strange plants can be found growing in large colonies in damp places especially streamsides.

Naming History

The large leaves were wrapped around butter to help keep it fresh, which gave the plant the common name of 'butterbur'. In addition Dioscorides, a Greek physician from Anazarbus in Cilicia, gave it the generic name of *Petasites* after the wide-brimmed hats called petasos. He was also the author of *De Materia Medica*, the most important and referred-to herbal for many centuries.

Folklore

Since a woman would depend on her husband, it was important for a girl to have some idea of whom she was likely to marry. Many forms of divination were used and a common one needed butterbur seeds. A young girl should rise early on a Friday morning, and sow the seeds before sunrise while chanting the words:

I sow, I sow,
Then come my own dear,
Come here, come here,
And mow and mow.

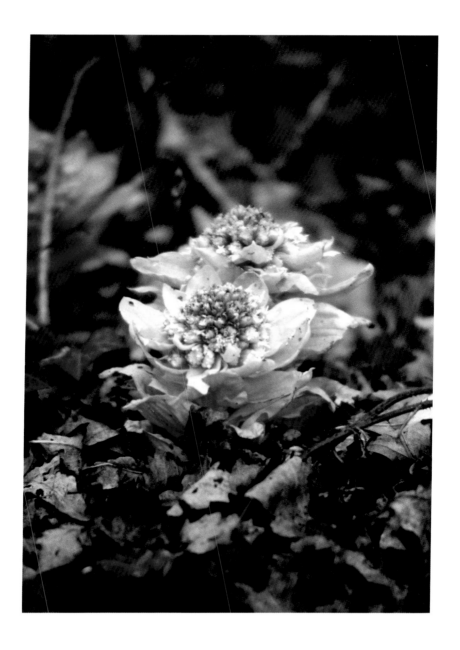

Butterbur

She should then in theory see a vision of her future husband mowing the meadow. If however she decided that she did not like the look of him, then the words 'have mercy on me' would make him disappear. It is not mentioned whether she got a second chance or not.

In the south of England, butterbur was considered poisonous. Somewhat illogically perhaps, children played happily amongst the leaves with the safe knowledge that no rats would brave the poison and come near them.

Other uses including medicinal

The dried roots of butterbur were supposed to be effective against 'the plague and pestilential fevers' by causing perspiration and making the patient 'sweat it out'. This may be related to the situation in Veryan Churchyard in Cornwall. Many plague victims were buried there and it was said that no plant would grow on the graves except butterbur, which thus earned the local name of plaguewort. In addition, the root, powdered and taken in wine, 'resisteth the force of any other poison'. Today the root is used as a heart tonic to stimulate the function of the heart.

Homeopaths make up a tincture of the root to treat headaches, neuralgia and inflammation of the urethra.

Burnet Rose
Rosa pimpinellifolia

Description

These very attractive roses grow as low bushes. The leaves are small and oval with serrated edges, very like those of a garden rose although smaller. They grow in pairs up the stem at frequent intervals. The pale cream to pink coloured flowers have a single ring of five petals, unlike the cultivated rose, and a central ring of yellow anthers. They appear during the months of May to July. Unlike the red hips produced in autumn by most roses, the fruits of the Burnet rose are purplish black.

Habitat

These plants are self supporting and grow in dry, open and exposed places, often coastal sand dunes.

Naming History

The Elizabethan botanist Gerard stated that this rose had leaves like the 'salad burnet', and gave it the name of 'burnet rose'. He also recorded the first sighting of a burnet rose growing in England.

Although the names sound related, the burnet rose is not associated with the burnet moth family. Their caterpillars actually feed on bird's-foot trefoil and, in the case of the six spot burnet moth, on trefoils and clover.

Folklore

There are a few local names given to the burnet rose which include 'cant-robin' from Fife, 'cat-rose' from Yorkshire and 'soldier's buttons' from Kirkcudbrightshire in Scotland. This latter name could be due to the shape of the flower, being likened to that of the cloth-covered buttons worn by the Elizabethan soldiers on their uniforms.

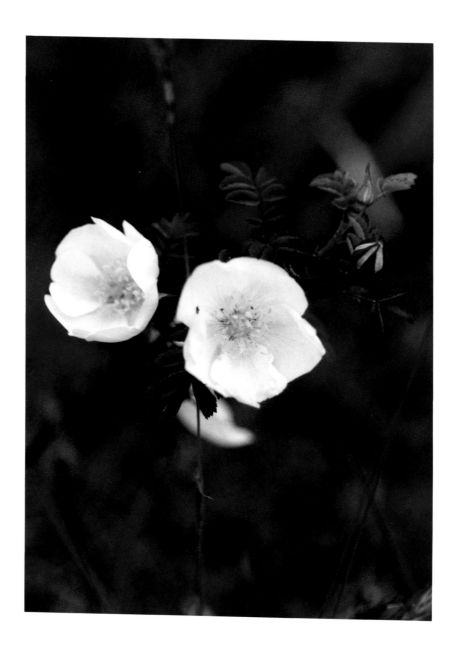

Burnet Rose

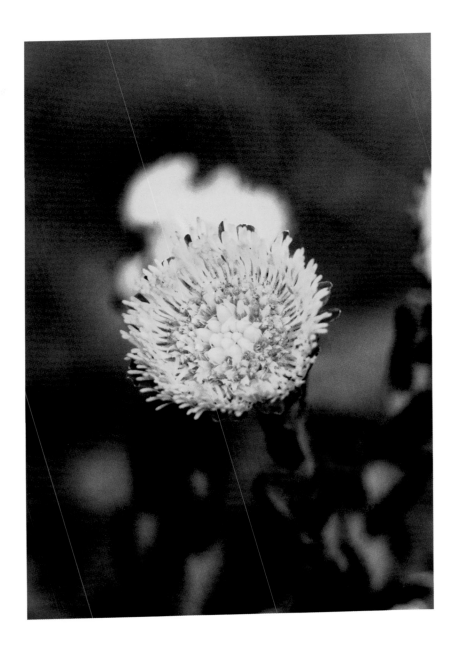

Coltsfoot

Coltsfoot
Troed yr Ebol, Carn yr Ebol
Tussilago farfara

Description

The flowers appear in February before the leaves. The single-headed flower consists of a ray of yellow bracts, like a daisy. They are solitary, set on stems covered with purplish scales. The leaves, which grow in large patches, are heart-shaped, 10 to 30cm across and have serrated edges. The undersides are grey and downy.

Habitat

This small attractive yellow flower is one of the first flowers of spring. It appears in early February on bare and waste ground, and flowers through until early April.

Naming History

The common name 'coltsfoot' comes from the shape of the leaves which bear a rather fanciful resemblance to a colt's hoof. This also gives rise to the Welsh name of 'Troed yr ebol', which translates to 'the foot of a foal (colt)'. These leaves also give the plant its country name 'son before the father', because the flowers appear before the leaves. The generic name *Tussilago* comes from the Greek word for cough, *tussis*, because for a long time this plant has been successfully used in the treatment of coughs and pulmonary complaints in general. The specific name *farfara*, is the Greek name for the white poplar, because the leaves look similar to those of this tree.

Folklore

Welsh country people say that if the seeds blow away when there is no wind, it is a sure sign of rain, and in the Scottish Highlands housewives gather the downy seeds to stuff cushions.

Other uses including medicinal

Coltsfoot was used in cough medicines and to relieve asthma as this old Welsh recipe demonstrates:

1) Put 2 pints of water in a large saucepan and add a handful of coltsfoot leaves (considering the size of a leaf one would probably be enough)
2) Boil until only half of the original water is remaining
3) Filter the infusion and add honey and a slice of lemon
4) Take 1 tablespoon three times a day until feeling better

Another use for the leaves was to be dried and then to be used as herbal tobacco, though whether this is any less injurious than ordinary tobacco is debatable. Pectoral beers, wine and jellies have been made from these leaves, which come up large and downy after the naked flowers have died back, and in Paris, a picture of a coltsfoot flower was used to advertise a pharmacy.

In the time before matches, when tinder boxes were used, the soft down from the leaves was used as tinder. In 1694 the author of the *Complete Herbal*, John Pechey, wrote that it was "wrapped in a rag, and boyl'd in a little lee, adding a little Salt-Petre, and after dried in the sun". For a long time, this type of tinder was popular in the Scottish Highlands.

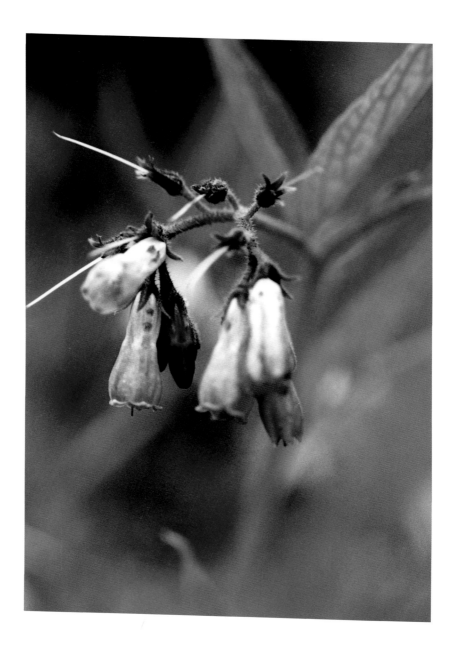

Comfrey

Comfrey
Llysiau'r Cwlwm
Symphytum officinale

Description

Comfrey is a tall, striking, but frequently overlooked plant. The broad, slightly hairy leaves, not unlike those of the foxglove, grow in great tufts, often near water. The creamy white or mauve bell-like flowers grow in clusters and usually appear in the early summer.

Habitat

Comfrey can most commonly be found growing in damp grassy areas, such as wet meadows, moorland, damp pastures, river banks and wet woods. It is widespread and can be found over most of Europe.

Naming History

Comfrey gets its name from the Latin *confirmo*, 'I strengthen', or *confero*, meaning 'I gather together', because people used this plant in the early treatment of fractures. In fact an old country name for comfrey is 'knitbone'. This plant was extensively used in medicine, hence the generic name *Symphytum* which comes from the Greek *symphyo*, 'I make whole', and *phyton*, meaning plant, while the specific name *officinale* shows it could be obtained from the apothecary.

The Welsh name 'llysiau'r cwlwm' translates as 'herb of the knot', an allusion to the bone-mending properties and similar to the English 'knitbone'.

Other uses including medicinal

Comfrey was pulled up and the roots were beaten into a pulp, and then spread onto a strip of leather and applied to the affected area to ease the pain and hopefully mend the bone. Applied in the same way outwardly, the roots were also said to help heal flesh wounds and cuts. In fact when crops and grass were cut with a scythe, wounds inflicted with this tool were treated using a poultice made of comfrey roots, and were then forgotten about. Also an old remedy of tea, made from the juice squeezed out from the roots, was thought to be beneficial in treating the bringing up of blood and for treating internal ruptures.

Although a wild flower, Comfrey was grown for hundreds of years in gardens, presumably in order to be readily available in case of injury. It is good for fertilizing the soil, and it is a good idea to plant a mixture of comfrey, tansy, yarrow and llysiau cadwgan (valerian) on your compost heap; in six weeks you will have excellent compost. In the seventeenth century, when many people were emigrating to North America, Comfrey was taken as one of the necessities of life, and has since established itself in the wild in New England.

Common Poppy
Pabi Coch, Llygad y Bwgan
Papaver rhoeas

Description

The common poppy is a familiar orange-scarlet flower up to 100mm across, with an almost silky feel to the petals. They appear from June to October, above the slender saw-toothed leaves. The fruits appear as vase-shaped structures with a row of slits around the top, from which the small black seeds can be shaken.

Habitat

During the summer months, these handsome flowers add a splash of colour to disturbed ground, especially to our arable fields and roadside verges.

Naming History

The common poppy's name comes from the Anglo-Saxon 'papig' but no more is known of its meaning nor of the origin of the generic name *Papaver*. The specific name *rhoeas* means 'flowing', an indication of how the seeds flow and scatter in the wind, from the ripe seed pods and also how easily the petals fall when the flower is picked or touched.

Maidens picked poppy heads and placed them in their pockets. Their success in love was determined by how fresh the leaves and petals were when they took them out again. Equally courting couples would place a petal on the palm of one of their hands and strike it hard with the other. A good resounding 'pop', indicated a true relationship, and is possibly the origin of the name 'poppy'.

Folklore

Because of its opium content, the poppy is considered to be the plant of sleep and because of its abundant seeds, of fertility. In Greek mythology Demeter's lovely daughter Persephone was kidnapped by Hades, who took her to his kingdom in the underworld. Poor Demeter was devastated and searched everywhere for her daughter. Her grief affected the crops and in consequence Hypnos, the god of sleep, sent poppies to grow at her feet, to help to comfort her and lull her to sleep. Whilst Demeter slept, Zeus persuaded Hades to allow Persephone to return from the underworld every spring and live with her mother for half of the year. So while Persephone was living with her mother, the earth goddess was

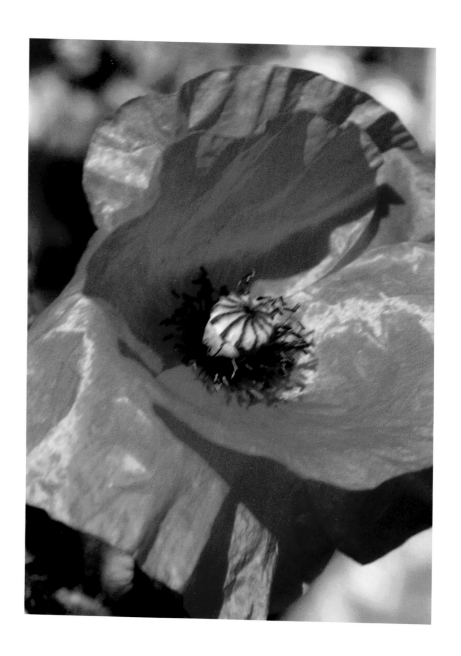

Common Poppy

happy and bestowed life and fertility back into the countryside. But when poor Persephone had to return back to the underworld for the winter, Demeter would be sad again and the earth would become hard and barren. Consequently the Greeks came to associate the poppy with renewal of life, regeneration and activity after sleep.

Every year on Armistice Day, 11th November, poppies are worn in remembrance of those who gave their lives during the First World War and subsequent wars. After the Battle of Flanders, poppies appeared in the fields. They were later adopted as a symbol by the British Legion and are now sold on Poppy Day in aid of ex-servicemen. The British Legion organised the first Poppy Day in 1921. Since then, millions of pounds have been raised for ex-servicemen and women and their dependants by selling artificial poppies.

There are many other old beliefs about poppies, the emblem of consolation and sleep. In Roman mythology, Morpheus the god of sleep was said to have given crowns of poppies to people that he wished to send to sleep. People thought that smelling poppies would induce a headache and held near the ear it could even cause earache! All this seems quite ridiculous, because the poppy can in fact cure a headache, earache, toothache and even insomnia. English country children thought that picking a bunch of poppies would bring on a thunderstorm, thereby giving the poppy some of its country names of 'thunderbolt', 'thundercup', 'thunder-flower' and 'lightning'. In the city of Liege in eastern Belgium, the poppy was considered as the '*fleur di tonit*', the 'thunder-flower' and picking it would generate a storm but, in contradiction to this, some people believed that placing poppies under the roof timbers of their houses kept away lightning.

These legends and tales belong properly to the familiar red poppy. In the west of Britain may also be found the yellow Welsh poppy *Meconopsis cambrica*. This is a true native of Wales, but may also be found growing in a few areas of south-west England, although it has been widely introduced elsewhere.

Other uses including medicinal

The seed and flowers were used to make a syrup to stop catarrh and mucus from head colds getting down into the stomach and lungs and causing further chest infections. It was also used to treat sore throats and loss of voice, and is still used today for similar purposes. An infusion of the petals is useful in treating asthma, bronchitis, catarrh, whooping cough and angina.

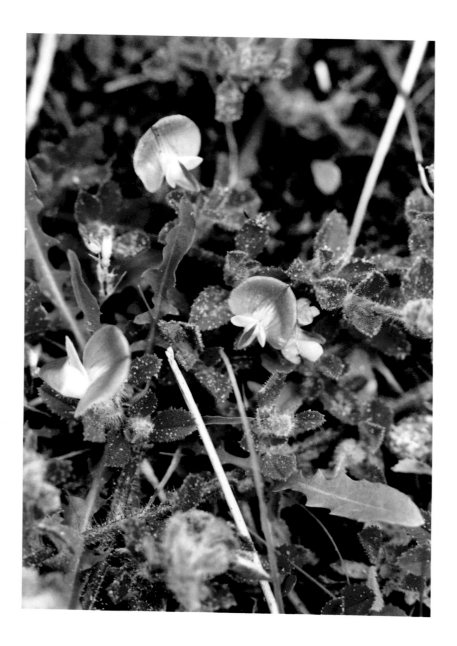

Common Restharrow

Common Restharrow
Tag yr Aradr
Ononis repens

Description

Restharrow is a short, low-growing plant, often found as an understorey to higher species. The stems are hairy, sometimes with soft spines, and the lipped pink flowers grow on leafy-stalked spikes from July to September in dry grassy places.

Naming History

The common name 'restharrow' came into use in the days before farms became mechanised, and the land was cultivated by using horses or oxen. The strong, matted roots would impede the progress of the plough or harrow through the soil. Although the farmers themselves did not appreciate this plant due to the extra effort that it caused to their ploughing, the animals certainly did. The generic name *Ononis*, comes from the Greek name *onos*, 'an ass', and *oninemi*, which means 'I delight'. There is an old belief which stated that farm animals loved to graze on the young shoots and to roll upon the plants' spines to scratch their backs. Children liked it too; they used to dig up the roots and chew them, saying that it tasted like liquorice. Hence some of the plant's other names of 'wild liquorice' and 'Spanish root', since liquorice was known as 'Spanish liquorice' or 'Spanish juice', or just 'Spanish' for short.

Folklore

English farmers certainly disliked restharrow for another reason. Although it was eaten with relish by the cows, it used to taint the taste of the milk, butter and cheese. and 'cammocky' butter was a nuisance in counties where restharrow is common.

Other uses including medicinal

An infusion of the root, particularly of the skin or bark, in wine was used as a diuretic and to break up and expel kidney stones, and was also believed to "open obstructions of the liver and spleen". The roots, when powdered, were also used to hasten the healing of skin ulcers. Modern herbalists use them for the same purpose and also for treating dropsy and cystitis. An infusion of the dried flowers is used to treat mouth infections.

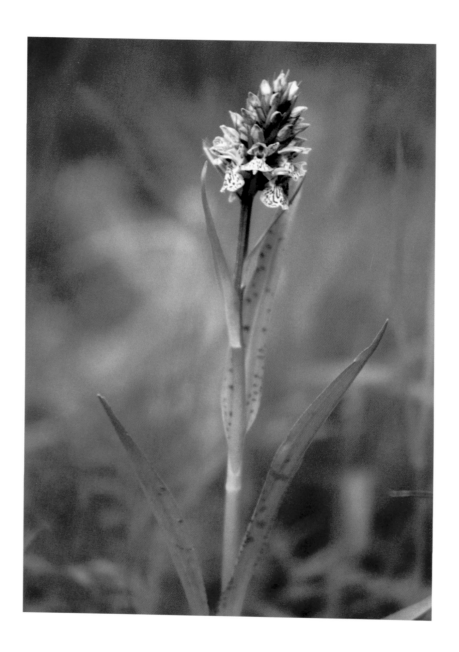

Common Spotted Orchid

Common Spotted Orchid
Tegeirian Mannog
Dactylorhiza fuchsii

Description
The flowers of this short to medium tall perennial are a pale pinky purple, dotted and lined with crimson or purple and with a very noticeable three-lobed lip. They appear during the summer months of June to August. The narrow lanceolate leaves are also darkly spotted.

Habitat
Common spotted orchids particularly favour a lime or alkaline soil. They can be found flowering in grassy places, open scrub and quite often near water.

Naming History
The common name 'orchid' comes from the Greek *orchis* 'testicle', an allusion to the double tubers of many species. William Turner called common spotted orchids 'hand satyrion' or royal satyrion. In 1548 he wrote that "'royal satyrion' or 'finger orchis' is called after the Latines *Palma Christi*, because it has large roots which are knobbed, not bulbed as the others, but branched or cut into sundrie sections like a hand". Indeed the 'dead men's fingers' of *Hamlet* may refer to common spotted and marsh orchids:

> There with fantastic garlands did she come
> of crow flowers; nettles; daises and long purples.
> That liberal shepherds give a grosser name,
> But our cold maids do dead men's fingers call them.

There are some very attractive local names for common spotted orchid. Some of these include; 'curlie-daddie' ('curly head') from Somerset, 'dead man's hand', also from Somerset and 'old women's pincushion' from Derbyshire.

Folklore
The common spotted orchid is sometimes called 'Gethsemane', from the legend that it was spotted by the blood of Christ. So perhaps some of these orchids were growing in the Garden of Gethsemane at the time of our Lord's agony.

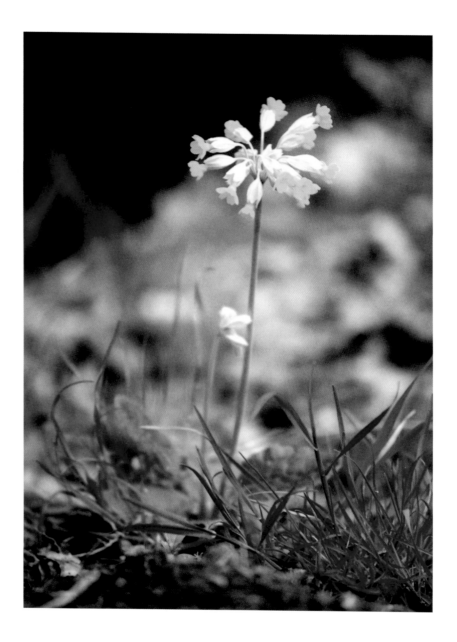

Cowslip

Cowslip
Briallu Mair
Primula veris

Description
In early spring clusters or rosettes of thick, slightly wrinkled, leathery leaves may be seen in grassy places. In March a flower stem sprouts upwards from the centre supporting a number of yellow flowers, hanging partly downwards in an almost bell-like fashion. The flowers up to two centimetres across, are rather tubular in shape, with the anthers and pistil deeply hidden within the ring of petals. Like its close relative the primrose, the cowslip is a spring flower before the growth of other vegetation casts it into shade.

Habitat
Many older people will remember this flower growing in carpets in the fields. Sadly, that is now a rare sight, but cowslips may still be found, particularly where traditional methods of farming are still practised. Wood margins, oakwoods and meadows are also sites where they grow.

Naming History
Cowslip is actually a contraction of 'cow's lip', not 'cow slip' as is sometimes thought; cows are quite sure-footed creatures. The leaves have a crinkled texture not unlike the lip of a cow, and the flower often grows where cows graze. The generic name *Primula* is from the Latin *primus*, meaning first, referring to the plant's early flowering. Another name for cowslip was 'palsywort', because it was used to treat this disease.

Folklore
Cowslip used to be called 'herb Peter' or 'St Peter's keys of heaven'. This was because the cluster of nodding flowers resembled a bunch of keys, which is the badge of St Peter. A legend from northern Europe tells a story about St Peter who, when he was told that a duplicate set of keys to the gates of heaven had been made, was so shocked that he dropped his own bunch. Where the keys fell, a cowslip grew. Whether St Peter ever found his keys or whether he had to use the spares was not told.

During the nineteenth and the beginning of the twentieth centuries, girls would use cowslips for divination. They picked bunches of them and wove them into balls, they would then play catch with each other singing:

> Tisty tosty, tell me true,
> Who shall I be married to.

While they were singing they would recite all the names of the local bachelors, and the last name sung before the ball landed on the ground ran the risk of becoming one of the girls' future husband. This was undoubtedly open to manipulation.

An ancient custom survived in Horncastle, Lincolnshire where, as late as 1805, cowslips were always strewn around the Maypole. Cowslips are now a protected species, so this could not happen any more.

Other uses including medicinal

The cowslip was considered a very useful herb indeed. The flowers alone were used as remedies for such conditions as vertigo, nightmares, false apparitions, frenzies, falling-sickness, palsies, convulsions, cramps and nerve pains. The roots eased back pain and bladder and urinary problems.

Nowadays the flowers are used for their sedative and anti-spasmodic properties. Dried and made into a tea they will ease insomnia, especially if made into a tincture and used in combination with hops and *Passiflora* (Passion flower). The flowers can also be made into an ointment, and applied to relieve sunburn.

Cuckoo Flower (Lady's Smock)
Blodyn y Gwcw
Cardamine pratensis

Description

The broad, bright green root leaves facing each other form a rosette around the base of the stem. The stem leaves are dissimilar, being lighter and more feathery in appearance. The four-petalled, white to pale lilac flowers with yellow anthers, appear in clusters at the top of an unbranched stem between the months of April to June.

Habitat

This delicately attractive perennial can be found growing in damp grassy places. It grows together in clusters, and often carpets damp water meadows, roadside ditches and verges and even woodland margins.

Naming History

The common name 'cuckoo flower' was almost certainly applied because this plant's flowering time coincides with the arrival of the cuckoo and the time it is first heard. The other name 'lady's smock' probably derived from the resemblance of the flowers to little smocks hanging out to dry in the wind and the fact that this is a spring flower much associated with milkmaids (an alternative name for this plant), and their smocks. The name smock seems to have come from the early English name 'lustmoce' and the name 'smick' more commonly used as 'smicket', came from the old name 'smick-smock' which was another name for a smock. Unfortunately, 'smickering' or to 'smicker' were words used to describe lecherous looks and purposes.

The generic name *Cardamine* comes from the Greek *kardamon* which means watercress, due to its similar taste. At one time this species was used as a heart sedative and its name derives from the Greek *kardia*, meaning 'heart', and *damao* 'subdue'. The specific name *pratensis* simply means that this plant grows in meadows.

Folklore

Cuckoo flower has also been called 'cuckoo spit flower', because although the white froth is made by the developing embryo of the shield bug, it used to be believed that cuckoos flying overhead spat on the plant below making it unlucky.

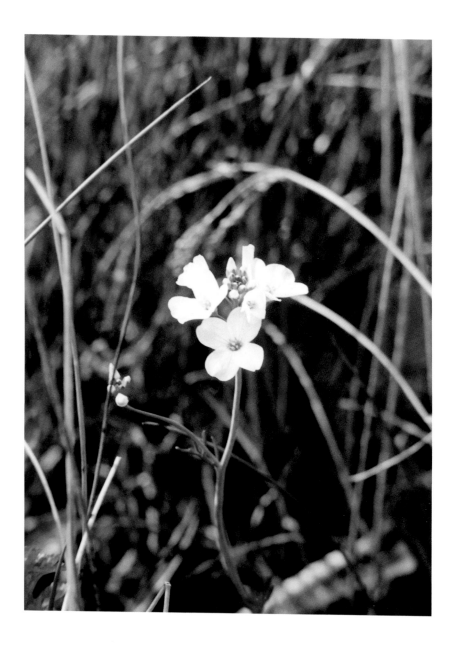

Cuckoo Flower (Lady's Smock)

The flower was also associated with fairies of evil disposition, and because of this, lady's smock was not included in such decorations as Mayday garlands, neither was it ever brought into the house.

William Shakespeare was almost certainly referring to lady's smocks when he wrote his famous line from *Love's Labour's Lost*, 'lady-smocks all silver white', and in a fifteenth or sixteenth-century Irish poem, cuckoo flowers are mentioned together with carefree young girls:

> Tender cress and cuckoo-flower,
> And curly-haired, fair-headed maids
> Sweet was the sound of their singing.

Other uses including medicinal

The cuckoo flower was described by Culpeper as being dominated by the moon. He said it was good for combating the symptoms of scurvy and was an excellent tonic, especially in cases where the appetite was lost. It has also been used in the treatment of epilepsy.

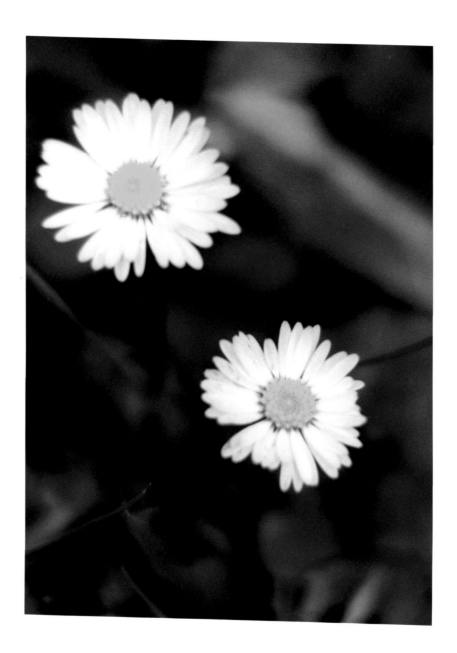

Daisy

Daisy
Llygad y Dydd
Bellis perennis

Description

Daisies must be familiar to everyone, especially those who made daisy chains in their childhood and those who cultivate lawns in later life. The spoon-shaped, slightly toothed leaves have a fuzzy surface and grow from a basal rosette. The solitary flowers consist of a yellow centre of disc florets, surrounded by many white florets that are sometimes tipped with red. They seldom grow to a great stature remaining at four inches (10cm) high or less.

A Welsh poet described the daisy as 'Deial aur rhwng dail arian', which translates to 'A golden dial between silver leaves'.

Habitat

Other than on lawns, daisies can be found on short turf almost anywhere. Being low-growing flowers, they cannot grow successfully in an environment of tall grass.

Naming History

The name daisy comes from the Saxon word *daeges-eage* meaning 'eye of day', because these flowers open in the morning to get the sunlight and close again in the evening. The Welsh name 'Llygad y dydd' means exactly the same. The generic name *Bellis* may come from the Latin *bella*, which means 'pretty' although the plant's usefulness as a wound herb makes it rather more likely that it comes from the Latin *bellum*, meaning 'war'. Daisies were also sometimes called 'bruisewort', because they were used to treat bruises. This name is also thought to have come from the Scottish name 'bairnwort', the 'baby's flower', because of its use in treating children's ailments and the fun that children have in making daisy chains.

Folklore

Daisies were, and still may be, used in divination. A young girl wanting to know if her love was requited, would pull the petals one by one from a daisy reciting 'he loves me, he loves me not,' until the last petal answered her query. Sometimes when a women had many suitors and could not decide whom she loved, she wore a daisy chain around her head. She would have plucked the petals from the flower beforehand, saying 'he loves me, he loves me not', thereby letting the flower decide for her. Equally if a girl picked a bunch of daisies with her eyes shut, the number of flowers she held in her hand when she reopened her eyes, was the number of years until she married.

Another story, though not about divinaton, is that the red tips on the petals of a daisy are caused by fairies dancing around the perimeter of the flower at night. They dance so hard that they make their feet bleed, leaving little red tips to the daisy's petals. Another legend is that the white daisies that grew at the base of Christ's cross were said to have grown from the tears of Mary Magdalene, and turned pink when spattered by His blood.

Other uses including medicinal

Country folk used to believe that if a child wore a daisy chain around its neck, it would protect it from being kidnapped by fairies. But if a child touched a daisy before it was weaned, it would be stunted. However, this belief was of advantage in days when people used to feed daisy roots to unweaned puppies to ensure that they did not reach maturity, as a way of coping with the problem of large and unwanted litters. Although the daisy's main use in past times was as a wound herb, it was also prescribed for stiff neck and lumbago. It was also said that chewing the fresh leaves helped to cure mouth ulcers!

The Welsh found the leaves extremely useful. As an infusion, either with or without milk, drunk three times a day, it would lower a fever. Alternatively the leaves were pounded and added to old lard to make a cream which would ease bruising and general aches and pains.

Dandelion
Dant y Llew
Taraxacum officinale

Description

The solitary flowerhead grows on a tall, thick fleshy stem, which exudes a sticky juice when snapped, from a basal rosette of deeply notched leaves, which can be picked and eaten in salads. The flower itself can measure up to 35-50mm across and comprises many bright yellow florets supported by green sepal-like bracts, often curving downwards. Each floret is a complete flower in itself, tubular in shape with the stamens and nectaries deep inside. There may be a hundred or more florets tightly packed together to form the composite flower, thus giving rise to the name of the group to which this species belongs, the *compositae*. After the flowers have been pollinated the petals fall and the developing seeds produce the familiar fluffy parachutes to form the seedhead known for generations as the 'dandelion clock'. The sight of dandelion seeds blowing across a field on a windy day, makes it clear how efficient this plant is.

Habitat

Dandelions can be found flowering throughout the year, but they appear at their best between the months of April to June. They especially like a lime soil and are in fact one of the commonest of field and wayside weeds. Dandelions will grow on almost any grassy or waste area and will even grow enthusiastically in your garden, although they have a very long taproot and are extremely difficult to remove, as gardeners know to their cost.

Naming History

The word dandelion, which is the common name for this well known garden weed, actually came from the French word *dent-de-lion*, meaning 'lion's tooth'. This could perhaps be due to the jagged edges of the leaves, which do look rather like lion's teeth, or possibly refers to the shape of the tap-root or the flower's florets. Another suggestion is that the lion was regarded as a symbol of the sun, and the dandelion flower does look very sunlike. The generic name *Taraxacum* may have come from the Arabic *talkh chakok* meaning bitter plant. If you bite a dandelion's stem it tastes very bitter, unlike the leaves which are sometimes used in salads.

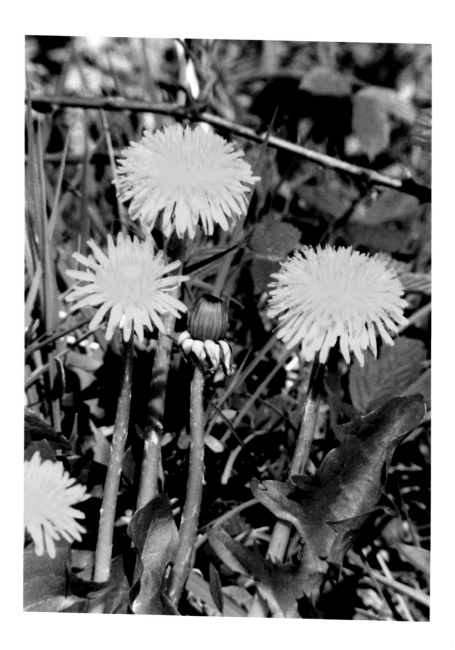

Dandelion

Folklore

For generations children have loved blowing the seeds from the dandelion 'clocks' to tell the time, each puff of breath supposedly representing an hour, until all the seeds have blown away. An old tale, perhaps the origin of this, says that if a child blows away all the seeds, his mother will reject him, so he should run home quickly if only a few seeds remain, to prevent this from happening.

In common with some other flowers, dandelion is connected with St John, perhaps because St John's Day falls close to midsummer. If witches were abroad at this time and plaguing country folk, dandelions picked on St John's Eve and placed on windowsills and over doorways would act as an effective repellent. The reason for this is unclear, but since witches exploited the powers of darkness, the bright flowers of dandelion may have symbolised the sun.

Other uses including medicinal

Due to its many healing properties one Welsh author described the dandelion as a 'little weed with a heart of gold'. The Welsh also made use of the roots from dandelions. By boiling an ounce of crushed roots with a pint of water for twenty minutes they created a tincture which was used for many ailments. By sieving the concoction and drinking it twice a day it could help with easing rheumatism (crydcymalau). Jaundice (clefyd melyn) and kidney stones (grafel) were also treated with the juice, which had the additional properties of reducing fever and was beneficial for skin complaints. The regular drinker of dandelion juice would be bright eyed and clear of complexion. The therapeutic properties were referred to in the *Herbal* written by the Physicians of Myddfai.

Dandelion has a strong diuretic effect and is used today in the treatment of a number of conditions, including water retention and hypertension. In time of shortage and during the wars, dandelion roots were sometimes ground up and used as a coffee substitute. This was also thought to relieve an upset stomach. The recipe for dandelion coffee was as follows:

1)Collect some strong healthy roots then wash and dry them thoroughly

2) Bake in a fairly hot oven (I could not discover for how long)

3) Grate finely and use as a caffeine free alternative

Beware of trying this yourself, because of this plant's strong diuretic properties, which led to the old country name of 'Piss-a bed'!

Europeans discovered that dandelion leaves were a rich source of vitamins and minerals. As well as having four times more Vitamin C in them than a lettuce they also have a healthy dosage of calcium, sodium, potassium and sulphur. Due to this knowledge the French and the Germans used the young leaves in salads. The Welsh also seem to have known this as they used the leaves in sandwiches as a detoxic.

Dandelions give off a gas (ethylene) which inhibits the growth of other plants, and thus helps to prevent the dandelion being choked by grass or other competitors. Gardeners sometimes put this to good use by spreading dandelion seeds beneath fruit trees to stop pest species establishing themselves.

Devil's-Bit Scabious
Glaswenwyn, Tamaid y Cythraul
Succisa pratensis

Description

Devil's-bit scabious grows to about 61cm (two feet) high. The narrow, smooth, crinkled edged leaves grow in pairs on opposite sides of the stem. Each stem bears a rounded head comprised of many small florets of a blueish purple colouring, which can very occasionally be pink.

Habitat

The flowers appear from June to October, and may be found in ungrazed grassland. It thus has to compete with tall grasses, which accounts for its height.

Naming History

Both the common and scientific names for Devil's-bit scabious are very descriptive. A few related species were once used to treat a variety of skin complaints which gave rise to the common name 'scabious' which comes from the Latin *scabies* meaning 'itch'. The generic name *Succisa*, like the common name 'Devil's bit', refers to the shortened root because it derived from the Latin *succisum* which means 'broken off'. The specific name *pratensis,* as in a number of other plants, simply means 'meadow dwelling'.

Folklore

According to popular belief, the scabious plant used to have quite a long root, that could be used for curing almost all diseases, but according to the *Great Herbal* of 1526 the Devil, who grudged man having such a useful medicine, bit it off short. The fifteenth century *Ortus Saniatis* told another version of the story in which the Devil attempted to use the root to give him excessive power, but the Virgin Mary intervened and put an end to his plan. In his irritation the Devil bit off the root.

Another superstition which arose in Cornwall was that folk should never pick a Devil's-bit scabious or Devil's button, because they feared that if they did the Devil would come and visit their bedside at night.

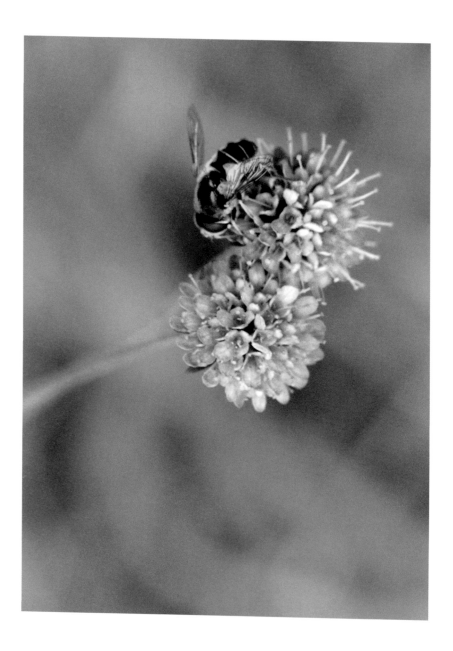

Devil's-Bit Scabious

Other uses including medicinal

The root of the herb was used as one of the kinder cures for the plague. It was boiled in wine and then drunk as a powerful relief to pestilence and poisons. Culpeper believed that beating the herb or root and then applying it externally to bruising, healed any internal bleeding by breaking down the blood clots which are formed. Also the juice taken from the herb was an effective cure for wounds in general.

To help reduce swelling and tumours in the throat a decoction of the herb made with honey of roses was used as a gargle. Adding powdered root to a beverage and drinking it helped to dispel worms from the body.

Although this herb is not currently prescribed by herbalists, until recently it was used to cure fevers and inflammatory diseases. An infusion of the herb aided the reduction of temperature naturally and helped to sweat out toxic substances.

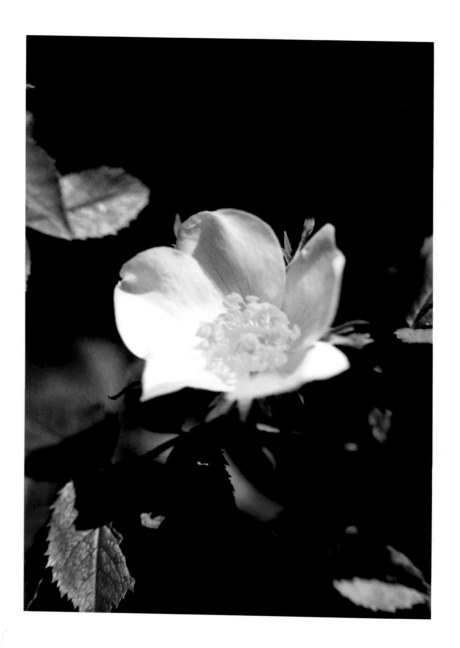

Dog Rose

Dog Rose
Rhosyn Gwyllt
Rosa canina

Description

Dog rose is a thorny climbing bush which entwines itself into British hedgerows. Unlike some other species of rose the dog rose can be recognised by its small curved thorns and arching stems. The small dark green oval leaves with serrated edges grow opposite each other in two or three pairs on a short stem. The pale pink to white, five-petalled flowers appear during the summer months of June and July. In the autumn they are replaced by the attractive bright red berries that we call rose hips.

Habitat

Dog rose or wild rose is a common and welcome sight in hedgerows during the summer months throughout the northern hemisphere.

Naming History

The name 'dog rose' originally came from the Roman naturalist Pliny. He said a Roman soldier used the root of the plant to cure himself of hydrophobia (a symptom of rabies), after being bitten by a mad dog. This gave rise to an early medicinal use in treating people with rabies. Hence the scientific name *Rosa canina*.

Folklore

The Tudor Rose came from the single, five-petalled dog rose. After the death of Henry VI, Henry of Richmond (1457-1509), son of Edmund Tudor, Earl of Richmond, and head of the House of Lancaster, adopted the red rose to emphasise Lancastrian claims. After his victory at the Battle of Bosworth in 1485 he was crowned King Henry VII and married Princess Elizabeth of York. The union gave rise to the Tudor Rose, a superimposition of the white rose, the emblem of York, on the red.

To many people the dog rose is symbolic of the English countryside as typified by G. K. Chesterton's poem 'The Rolling English Road':

The wild rose was above him when we found him in the ditch.

Other uses including medicinal

Dog rose frequently has a reddish-yellow gall growing on the tip of the stem. These are called 'briar balls' or sometimes 'robin's pincushion', and they are made by the gall wasp *Rhodites rosae*. At one time these briar balls were collected and sold by the apothecaries. They were powdered and a decoction of the powder was taken as a diuretic to break kidney stones and for colic. The larva that the briar ball contained was regarded as an additional bonus. This was also dried and ground into a powder. It was then diluted and drunk to kill and expel worms from the belly. It was also an old custom for country people to hang briar balls around their necks to guard themselves against whooping cough.

Children used to love using the seeds from rose hips as itching powder, they used to push them down each others necks, thus giving them the country names of 'buckie-lice' in Scotland and 'tickling Tommies' in Devon. Rose hips were used in making commercial rose hip syrup, making them the last of the wild crops to be picked from the hedgerows by hand, mostly by children who were paid by the quantity they gathered. Not only do they look pretty in the autumn hedgerows, they are a very necessary food supplement for the birds in winter.

Dog Violet
Fioled y Ci, Sanau'r Gwcw, Gwiolydd Gyffredin
Viola riviniana

Description

The leaves of dog violet are heart-shaped and deeply veined. Each leaf grows on a separate stalk, all of which rise from the base of the plant. They appear in spring before the flowers. These are 15-25mm across with five petals, one of which forms a large downwards-pointing lip. Despite giving its name to the colour violet, the flowers vary greatly in hue, from deep purple to pale pink. Like the leaves, each flower grows on a single stem.

Habitat

Dog violets are spring flowers, visible from March to May. They flourish in grassy places, hedgerows and woods before they are shaded out by the long grass and leaf canopy of summer.

Naming History

The name 'violet' came from the French, but before this name came into use, violets were given cuckoo names, such as 'cuckoo's shoe' in Cheshire, 'cuckoo's stockings' in Shropshire and 'sanau'r gwcw' (cuckoo's socks) in Wales. Many wild flower names were given the prefix 'cuckoo', because they are in flower around the time that the cuckoo is first heard. In Ireland they are called *salchuach*, 'cuckoo's heel', because the spur of the flower is thought to resemble a cuckoo's foot. The term 'dog' is often used to indicate that the plant is a smaller variety than the common or cultivated version, for example 'dog rose', which is smaller than the garden rose.

Ion is the Greek name for violet, possibly because Io is said to have fed on violets when she was transformed by Jupiter into a heifer, or perhaps after some nymphs of Ionia who presented a bunch of violets to Zeus, the father of the gods.

Folklore

Like the snowdrop and primrose, violets had the reputation of being unlucky if gathered in small numbers, and if a few were brought into the house, you might well have found that your hens stopped laying. Unfortunately there seems to be no record of what number constitutes 'a few', and it is not clear what would have

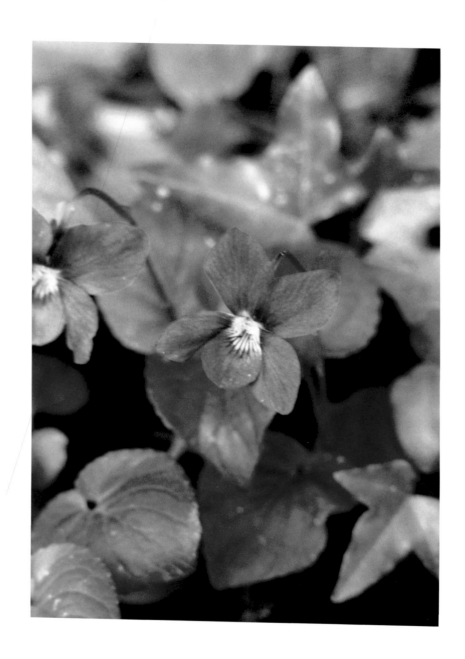

Dog Violet

happened to your hens if you gathered a large number. Violets blooming in the autumn indicated an epidemic or even death, but dreaming about them indicated increased wealth (presumably winning the lottery these days). In Gloucestershire people refused to bring violets into the house, on the ground that they harboured fleas, but worn as a wreath around the neck they were said to help to prevent drunkenness.

The violet is a flower which is usually taken as the symbol of modesty, but fabled by the ancients to have sprung from the blood of the boaster Ajax. A hero of the Trojan War, Ajax was the son of Telemon and King of Salamis. He was a big man, daring but slow-witted. He killed himself when the armour of Achilles was awarded to Ulysses as champion, and not to him. Shakespeare sticks to the old tradition that this flower was raised from the body of Io, by the agency of Diana, and quotes in his play *Hamlet*:

> Lay her in the earth,
> And from her fair and unpolluted flesh
> May violets spring.

The poet William Wordsworth wrote about them saying:

> Long as there are violets
> They will have a place in story.

In colloquial French, the flower means 'think of me' and that is why it is so often used as a symbol of love. On one occasion in history, this meaning acquired a different association. After the first defeat of Napoleon Bonaparte in 1813, the exiled Emperor rallied his followers with the declaration:

> I will return to France when the violets bloom in Springtime.

The loyal Bonapartists adopted the flower as their emblem, meaning that they were thinking of Napoleon, and true to his promise Napoleon returned from Elba in temporary triumph to Paris in March 1815. Unfortunately for him, Wellington heard about it too... As a consequence of Napoleon's defeat, the Bourbon monarchy banned the wearing of the violet as a seditious symbol.

Other uses including medicinal

Violets are still used today to fragrance perfume, and as a flavouring for sweetmeats as well as for declarations of love in posies. The mauve colour of violets is an indication of the love of truth and the truth of love. In the *Language of Flowers*, the white violet is an emblem of innocence, and the mauve violet of faithful love.

It was said that the leaves could help to cure cancer, strengthen the heart and quieten the nerves. In Wales a treacle was made from the flowers which was regarded as being unrivalled at curing colds, coughs and chest complaints:

½ lb of violet flowers
1¼ pints of boiling water
lump sugar

1) Add the violet flowers to the boiling water and leave the mixture for 4 hours 20 minutes
2) Filter the juice and add two times the amount of sugar as the liquid's weight (roughly 4lb!)
3) Place mixture on the fire but do not allow to boil
4) Bottle the treacle and use when needed

It does not say how long it took to collect half a pound of violet petals, but the gatherer would have been occupied for quite some time!

Enchanter's Nightshade
Llysiau Steffan, Llysiau'r Swynwr
Circaea lutetiana

Description

Although relatively common, enchanter's nightshade is an inconspicuous plant. The slender stem, up to about 50cm tall, carries oval pointed leaves in pairs at regular intervals. The stem extends above the leaves to form the flowerspike, bearing pairs of tiny (5mm) two-petalled white flowers. These bloom first at the bottom of the spike, which continues to grow upwards as more flowers open. The lower ones become small hooked fruits before the upper ones do, the hooks being used to catch in the fur of animals or trousers of walkers to disperse the seeds.

Habitat

Enchanter's nightshade prefers woods and shady places, where it forms sometimes quite dense patches. It is a summer-flowering plant, blooming from June to September, and fruiting throughout most of that period.

Naming History

This plant received both its common and generic names from Circe, or Kirke, who was an enchantress from Greek mythology. It was said that the seeds catch in the clothes of folk brushing past, as easily as Circe could have ensnared them with her spells. The name was also shared with the mandrake plant, which was also classified as a 'nightshade' and was used in magic; and not surprisingly the two names became mixed. The specific name *lutetiana* means 'from Paris'. Lutetia having been the ancient name of this city, although some other French names also include '*herbe a la magicienne*', '*enchanteresse*', '*herbe aux sorciers*' and rather more Christian sounding, '*herbe de Saint-Simon*' and '*herbe de Saint-Etienne*'.

Enchanter's nightshade was known to the Anglo-Saxons as 'Aelfthone' and was used by them as a medicine to counteract 'elf-sickness'. Elf-sickness is almost certainly the same affliction as 'elf-shot', an unknown disease which was supposed to be caused by an elf-arrow.

Some other country names include 'dragon-root' from Ireland, 'philtrewort' from Yorkshire and 'witch-flower' from Somerset.

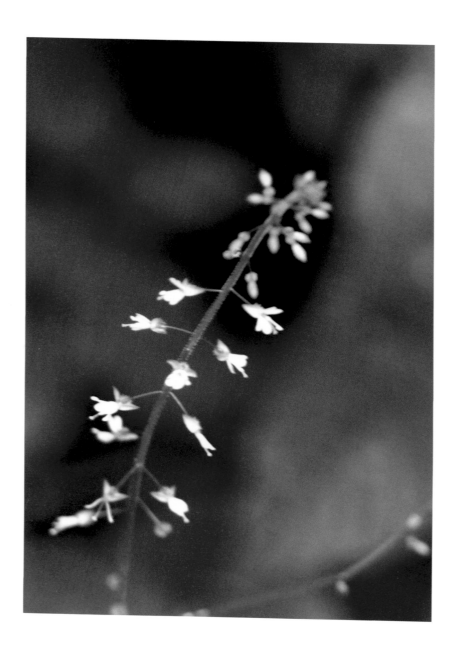

Enchanter's Nightshade

Folklore

Circe was an enchantress who lived on the Greek island of Aea, and was said to transform all who drank of her cup into swine. When Ulysses landed there, on his rather extended way home from the Trojan war, Circe transformed all his sailors into swine. The wily Ulysses resisted this metamorphosis by adding a herb called 'Moly' (wild garlic), which had been given him by Hermes, to his wine before he drank it. He drew his sword and threatened Circe to her bed. Later she came round to his point of view, his men were released and they continued on their way rejoicing:

> Who knows not Circe,
> The daughter of the sun, whose charmed cup,
> Whoever tasted lost his upright shape,
> And downward fell into a grovelling swine?
>
> John Milton

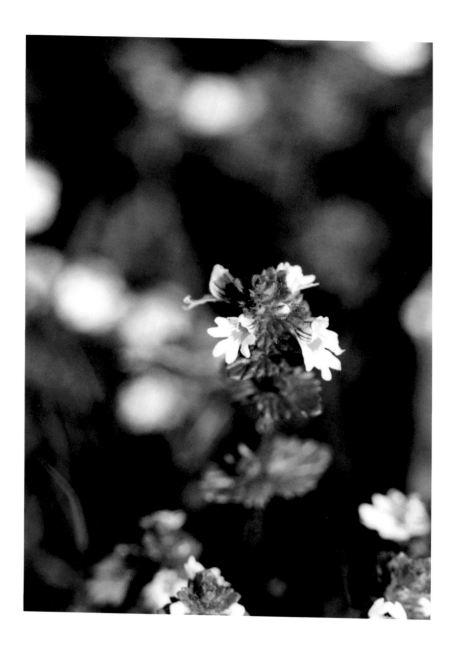

Eyebright

Eyebright
Effros, Golwg Christ, Llygad Christ, Llygad Siriol
Euphrasia officinalis

Description

This small, low-growing, creeping plant flowers from June to October. It is a semi-parasitic hairy annual and often well branched. The leaves are more or less oval, deeply toothed and grow opposite each other on the stem. It is a member of the figwort family and the characteristic small, two-lipped white flowers are often tinged violet or have purple veins with a yellow spot on the lower lip, which is three lobed.

Habitat

Eyebright can be found generally in grassy places, particularly where the over-all height of the grass is fairly low, such as mountainous areas and stabilised sand dunes.

Naming History

In past times eyebright was used as a cure for many eye diseases, which gave it its common and specific name of *officinalis*. Its generic name *Euphrasia* comes from the Greek *euphrasio*, 'delight', and was almost certainly adopted in recognition of the plant's use in curing blindness. In fact the Welsh have two attractive names for this plant. They are 'golwg Christ', 'Christ's sight', and 'llygad Christ', 'Christ's eye', a grateful indication of its value.

Folklore

John Milton in *Paradise Lost* (Book XI, 411) mentions how the Archangel anointed Adam's eyes with 'Euphrasie [Eyebright] and Rue and three drops of water from the Well of Life', to enable him to see death and thus the miserable future of mankind:

> Death thou hast seen
> In his first shape on man; but many shapes
> Of Death, and many are the wayes that lead
> To his grim Cave, all dismal.

Other uses including medicinal

During the Middle Ages and later, Eyebright was used by ladies for brightening their eyes, which they considered made them look more attractive. In fact William Coles wrote about it in his herbal *Adam in Eden* or *The Paradise of Plants* (1657): "The purple and yellow spots and stripes, doth very much resemble the diseases of the eyes, as blood-shot…" In 1694 John Pechey wrote down this recipe in *The Complete Herbal of Physical Plants*.

1½ oz of water of eyebright
1/2 oz of water of fennel
1oz of white rose-water
2 drams of prepared tutty (*zinc oxide*)
2 grains of camphire

"Mix them together and then drop two or three drops into the eye, warm, twice a day. This is good when the eye is much bruised."

Nicholas Culpeper also wrote about it in his *Complete Herbal* published in 1649. He said "the juice or distilled water of eyebright, taken inwardly in white wine or broth, or dropped into the eyes, helps all infirmities of the eyes that cause dimness of the sight. A conserve of the flowers has the same effect. It also helps a weak brain or memory." It appears that the Welsh had also heard of Culpeper's remedies as they used the plant in a similar way. The Welsh believed that drinking a tea made from the leaves morning and evening would strengthen the eyes.

Eyebright is still popularly used for treating eye infections today. No herbal dispensary is likely to be without it, and it is still used for treating inflammatory eye disease, conjunctivitis and other eye infections.

Field Forget-Me-Not
Glas y gors, N'ad fi'n angof
Myosotis arvensis

Description

Field forget-me-not is a medium tall annual. The texture of the leaves is softly hairy, like the feel of a mouse's ear. They are oblong and usually unstalked, clasping the stem, but are not opposite to each other. The lower leaves are stalked and form a rosette around the base of the stem. The five-petalled flowers are small, blue/grey in colour, but usually pink in bud with a yellow sepal tube in the centre. They appear in branched clusters at the top of the stems.

Habitat

Field forget-me-not, as the name suggests, grows in fields, particularly in dry soil conditions. Its height means that it can compete with grasses and other medium tall plants, and is usually seen in uncut meadows. It is not, for instance, found in close-cropped or sheep-nibbled turf. The flowers may be seen from April to October.

Naming History

The common name 'forget-me-not' originally belonged to the ground pine, a hairy plant and member of the labiate family. It has two-lipped yellow flowers marked with red spots, and smells of pine when crushed. The name apparently referred to the very unpleasant taste it left behind in the mouth. However early in the nineteenth century for some unknown reason, it became transferred to this little plant. The generic name *Myosotis* comes from the Greek *mys*, meaning 'mouse' and *ous*, 'ear' because the leaves resemble the soft, hairy texture of a mouse's ear. *Arvensis* simply means that it grows in fields.

Folklore

The forget-me-not was used as a symbol of great affection. Women used to wear a corsage or posy pinned on their bodice, and if it contained a forget-me-not, then they would not be forgotten by their lover. This was illustrated by the German tale of the knight, who bent and picked a bunch of forget-me-nots for his lady as they were both strolling beside a river. Unfortunately, the knight slipped and fell in. Before he was carried away by the current and drowned, he threw the flowers to his lady, crying out *'vergisz mein nicht!'* 'forget me not!'

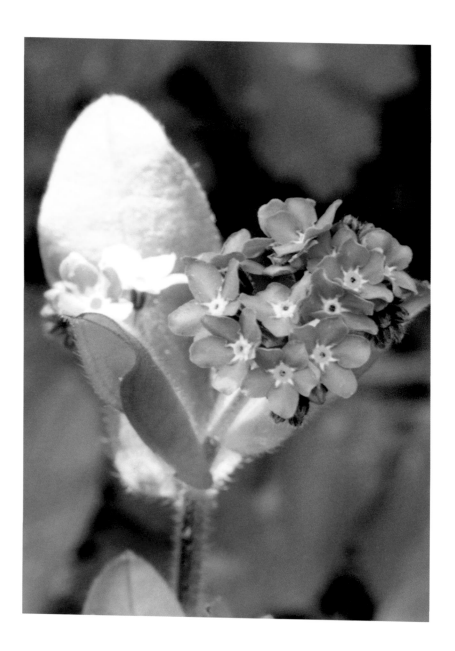

Field Forget-Me-Not

Other uses including medicinal

Forget-me-not was said to be useful for treating dog bites and even snake bites, and steel tempered with its juice was said to be hard enough to saw through stone.

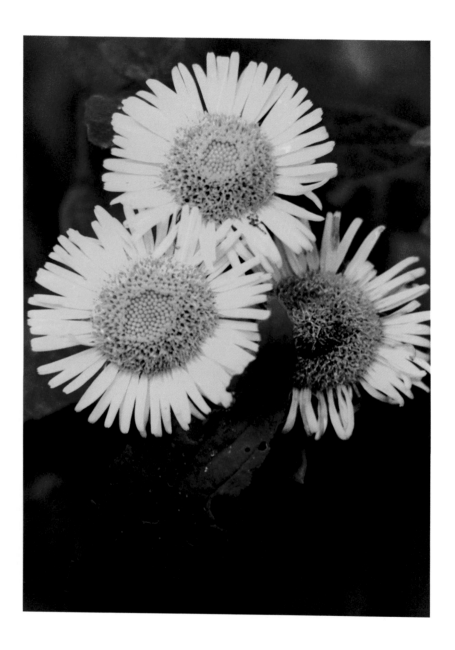

Fleabane

Fleabane
Amhrydlwyd, Chweinllys, Cedowydd
Pulicaria dysenterica

Description

Fleabane can grow up to about eight inches (20cm) in height. The leaves are lanceolate and wavy-edged with the base clasping the stem. They have a soapy smell when crushed, which makes this plant repulsive to animals. During the late summer months of July to September clusters of yellow flat-topped daisy-like flowers appear, these measure about 15-30mm across.

Habitat

Fleabane is found growing amongst long grass in damp marshy areas, such as wet meadows, ditches and hedgerows. It can form large communal patches.

Naming History

In Devon fleabane is known as the 'harvest flower', because it blooms during the harvest time. The common name 'fleabane' is a description of its uses. The word bane is Old English meaning to kill or destroy, and survives in the watered down version 'to banish', meaning to get rid of. The generic name *Pulicaria* simply means flea and *dysenterica* seems to be a reference to the effect (dysentery) that the plant has on these unfortunate creatures.

Other uses including medicinal

In the days when houses had earth or stone floors, people used to put down rushes as insulation and as a means to keep the floors clean. Anyway the rushes would have felt nicer to walk on. In the old farm houses the family would sleep at one end and the animals would sleep at the other, so fleas would have been rife. Therefore fleabane was strewn on the floor amongst the rushes to kill the fleas. It is assumed that it was the juice of the plant that was responsible for killing the fleas. However, seeing as the soapy smell of the leaves is so distasteful to other animals, maybe the fleas don't like it either.

Decoctions and infusions of the dried herb had an astringent action, and were used against dysentery; but the main use of this plant was as a flea repellent.

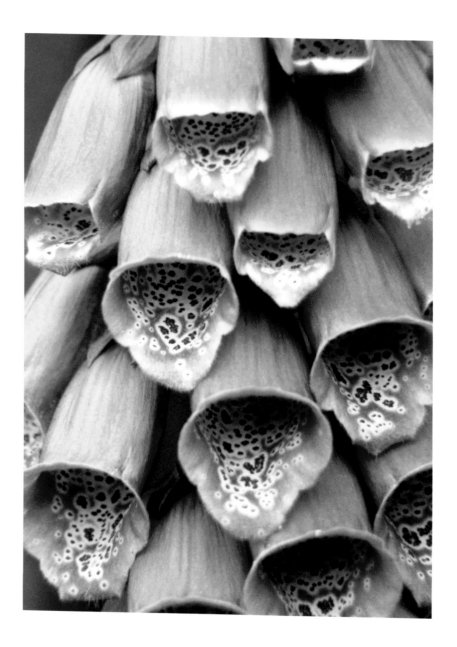

Foxglove

Foxglove
Bysedd y Cŵn, Ffion
Digitalis purpurea

Description

The spectacular foxglove is a familiar sight on banks and hedgerows. The conspicuous flower spike may be up to one and a half metres tall, supporting 20 or 30 bell shaped flowers. Each flower, mostly pink to purple, but sometimes paler or even white, has a lighter interior with dark spots. The lower flowers open first, followed by those further up as the spike grows, and seeds are produced in the same order. The flowers appear between June and September and are frequently pollinated by bumble bees. The leaves are large, soft and wrinkled, growing mainly from the base of the stem but also further up as the spike grows.

Habitat

This tall stately plant likes growing in damp and shady places, such as woods, scrubland and hillsides, usually on acid soils, though it is not uncommonly found in limestone areas as well. It is a very slow-growing plant and takes up to three years to mature before it flowers. In the autumn the flowers die back from the base of the flower spike forming the seeds. These then drop and germinate producing new young plants, and the old parent plant dies back.

Naming History

The common name of foxglove is probably a corruption from the Swedish 'folk's gloves' meaning fairyfolk, (who must have very large fingers), or it could have come from the Anglo-Saxon name 'foxes glew', 'fox-music', due to the bell-like flowers. Maybe they thought that a fox could ring the bells as it brushed past. Other country names include 'fairy's glove', 'fairy's cap', 'fairy's thimbles', 'witch's gloves', 'bloody fingers' and 'dead men's bells'. Some very attractive Welsh names for foxglove are 'gwyniadur Mair' (Mary's thimble),and 'menig Mair', (Mary's gloves). In Welsh there are at least two dozen flowers named after Mary, which shows what great devotion the Welsh country folk gave to the Virgin Mary. Other slightly more superstitious names include 'fenig y tylwyth teg', ('fairies' gloves'), and 'chlatsh y cwn', ('hit\strike the dog'). Whereas in Scotland they are called 'dead men's bells' and if you can hear them ringing, then you are not long for this world.

Folklore

There is an old country tale that says that once bad fairies gave the fox a foxglove, so that he could put the flowers on his toes and then stalk the hen houses in silence. In the Freiburg area of Switzerland, they call the foxglove 'Dey di diablho' or the 'Devil's thimble', so called because the Devil is said to have worn the flower petals on his fingers. But it had its good uses too; by providing hats to elves, refuges for fairies to hide in, and protecting mortals from fairies.

During the 1600s when many people feared witches, a woman was tried and found guilty of dealing with witchcraft and fairy folk. Her crime was to have killed a child by poisoning it with foxglove. More likely she was a healer who accidentally administered an incorrect dose resulting in the child's death.

The old belief that children could be kidnapped by fairies prompted this test to see if a child were a changeling. A foxglove bloom was pounded down and then three drops of the juice were put on the tongue and three in the child's ear. The child was then placed on a large shovel and swung three times in the doorway, while being challenged. If a fairy was present, it was then abjured to leave.

Other uses including medicinal

From the sixteenth century, foxgloves were used for treating sores, ulcers and flesh wounds. In the seventeenth century Italians used foxgloves to heal fresh wounds and cleanse old ones, hence the saying 'The Aralda or foxglove is a balm for every wound'. However it was not until the eighteenth century that its properties for treating heart problems were discovered. Dr Withering, the Warwickshire doctor who discovered digitalin as a treatment for heart disorders, first noticed its effect on the dropsical patients of a Shropshire wise woman and started experimenting. He published his findings in An account of the foxglove and some of its medical uses, in 1785. When he died in 1799 a foxglove was carved on his tombstone in the churchyard of Edgbaston Old Church. Dr Erasmus Darwin, grandfather of Charles Darwin, insisted on promoting the worth of digitalin, now called digitoxin, and taking the credit of the discovery onto himself, thus taking it away from Dr Withering. He was persuaded by his colleagues to record his discoveries, but naturally he could not do so without ruining his reputation. Instead he redeemed himself by naming a species of plant 'Witheringia' in memory of the doctor who discovered its worth.

In 1962 further research into the properties of digitalin led to the discovery that the drug can be used to treat glaucoma and the hereditary disease muscular dystrophy. Today foxgloves are farmed in large quantities and the leaves powdered for use in tablets. On the larger farms in Pennsylvania and other American states, enough foxgloves are grown to provide for 250,000,000 tablets a year.

Germander Speedwell
Llysiau Llywelyn, Llygad y Gath, Llygad Doli
Veronica chamaedrys

Description

The largest of the speedwell family, this very pretty plant can be recognised by its vivid blue flowers. These are small, about 10mm across, with four unequally-sized petals, and grow on short spikes arising from the base of the upper leaves. It grows in a sprawling or rambling fashion, with the pointed oval leaves growing in opposite pairs on very short stalks. The flowers can be seen from April to June.

Habitat

Germander speedwell is quite common, and grows generally in grassy places.

Naming History

In the sixteenth century, germander speedwell was called wilde germander, germander having descended through mediaeval Latin from the Greek *chaman-drua*, a corruption of *chamai*, meaning 'on the ground' probably referring to the way the plant spreads, and *drus,* which surprisingly enough means 'oak' in Latin, as if the speedwell or any other *chamaedrys* were a dwarf oak. In Cheshire germander speedwell is known as 'break-basin', since the petals fall very easily and may have a fanciful resemblance to broken china when lying on the ground. There is also a most attractive Welsh name – 'llygad doli', or 'dolly's eyes', because of the flower's resemblance to the bright blue eyes of a doll.

Folklore

'Speedwell' meant a plant of the roadside which 'speeds you well', so in Ireland speedwell used to be sewn into travellers' clothes to keep them safe when embarking on a journey. An alternative name for speedwell is 'bird's eye', but unfortunately this has some very unattractive stories attached to it. Children in Somerset were told, 'if you pick a bird's eye, birds will fly down and peck out your own eyes'. Equally to do this deed in Dorset meant your mother's eyes would be pecked out, or worse still in Devonshire, torn out. All these stories are illustrated by the West Country name for this little plant of 'pick-your-mother's-eyes-out'. The blue petals of germander speedwell or bird's eye tremble and fall very easily when touched, and will break your mother's heart. Symbolically the flowers of the germander speedwell are not only associated with birds, but to other evil persons as well, such as Robin Goodfellow or the Devil, and then in total contrast to the angels, God and Christ. So if a person destroys a flower, which could so easily happen, then revenge will be taken, although its exact form is not specified. In many cases the Christian church imposed its own symbolism on existing rituals and superstitions in order to remove pagan associations, and it is possible that that is what has happened here.

The following story helps to indicate the early discovery of speedwell's medicinal properties in Wales.

A shepherd noticed a stag who had been bitten on the hindquarters by a wolf. However, the stag partook of the herb and rolled in amongst the leaves whereupon his wound was healed. Another story tells of further properties belonging to the plant. Apparently a French king had been afflicted with leprosy for eight years and nothing had been an effective cure. But when some speedwell was brought to him, his malady left him.

In Germany people believed that picking speedwell would bring on a storm, which may indicate why in Northamptonshire it is called 'strike-fire', presumably because of the lightning, although the connection between Northamptonshire and Germany is not clear.

Other uses including medicinal

The leaves used to be sold in the London markets as a useful herb, whilst the Germans discovered that the leaves made a particularly good tea. The tea was at its most beneficial when made from fresh leaves and drunk daily. Women used to make a tincture from the leaves, and by drinking it often found a good cure for many ailments including; stomach wind, shortness of breath and coughs. It also appears to have been useful in reducing pain and was used to ease a headache and for back and kidney pain. This tincture was also used for dispelling toxins from the body by making the patient sweat.

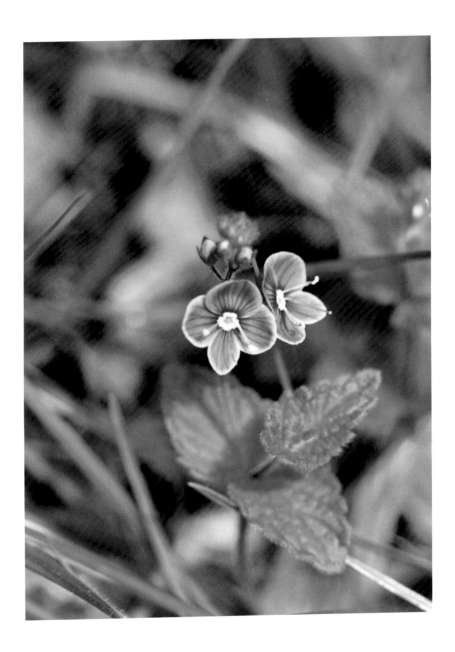

Germander Speedwell

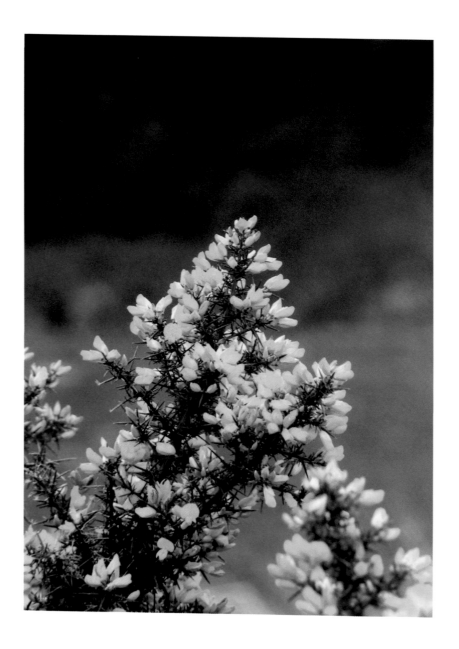

Gorse

Gorse
Eithin
Ulex europaeus

Description

This well known and heavily armed evergreen shrub is a member of the pea family. It grows in a tall and leggy fashion, shading out the ground beneath it. The rigid, furrowed and extremely sharp spines, that at first sight appear to be stems, are actually modified leaves. Like other evergreens, the leaves are not in fact everlasting, but are shed at no particular time at intervals of two to three years, forming a dense mat resembling dead pine needles under the bush, preventing the growth of other plants beneath. The characteristic pea-shaped flowers are a rich golden yellow and almond scented, and grow on leafy-stalked spikes. In due season the flowers give way to hard dry black seed pods that can be heard cracking open on a hot summer's day as the seeds are catapulted away from the parent bush.

Habitat

Gorse is very common and flowers all year round. It grows in dense patches on open hillsides and heaths, making bright yellow areas in times of maximum bloom.

Naming History

The name 'gorse' is probably descended from the Anglo-Saxon word '*gorst*' meaning 'a waste' because this shrub often grows in rough or waste places. Gorse is also known by the name of 'furze', which comes from another Anglo-Saxon word '*fyrs*', because people used it for firewood. *Ulex* has as unknown meaning, except that it was used by Pliny the Roman naturalist to describe a spiny shrub. The specific name *europaeus* means that this shrub grows in Europe.

Folklore

Long ago in Ireland it was believed that if you wore a sprig of furze it would prevent you from stumbling, and they hung furze flowers over their doorways on May Day to frighten away any witches and fairies. This custom was also carried out on the Isle of Anglesey.

Other uses including medicinal

Before the development of the coal trade, gorse was a very useful fuel. In the West Country every farm had its own 'vuzz' brake. After it was cut and faggoted the vuzz was then used to fire the 'cloam' or china clay ovens. After the spines had been well crushed, the gorse made valuable winter fodder for the animals. This crushing was often carried out in the cider mills.

The Romans used the stems and leaves of gorse bushes to filter the silt from their gold mines, trapping the gold dust. This technique was known as 'hydraulicking' or ground sluicing. A gentle flow of water was used to wash the silt through the filter beds which trapped the gold dust, allowing the rest of the silt to flow away. They tried many different filters, but gorse was one of the favourites.

Great Mullein
Clust y Fuwch, Pannog Melyn
Verbascum thapsus

Description

This tall and obvious plant may grow to two metres in height. It is covered with thick white woolly down, especially on the stem. The five-petalled flowers are bright yellow and up to 30mm across, growing in a spike at the top of the single stem. The leaves are broad and pointed. The flowers occur from June to August.

Habitat

Great mullein grows in dry places, mostly dry grassland and open scrub.

Naming History

This tall stately plant is sometimes called 'Aaron's rod', because the tall flower spike was likened to the staff carried by the biblical character. The common name mullein could have come from the French word 'moleine'. Moleine was a lung disease contracted by cattle, which could be treated by this plant. More likely it comes from the Old English word 'wolleyn' or 'wulleyn', meaning 'woollen' on account of the plant's soft velvety leaves. It was said that poor people used to place the thick woolly leaves inside their shoes for extra warmth.

Folklore

An old name for great mullein was the 'candlewick plant', because the down from its leaves was used in making tinder for tinder boxes and wicks, before cotton wicks for oil lamps were used. It used to have the less attractive name of 'hag's taper', too, because it was said that witches liked using the leafy down in their lamps, and as an ingredient in sorcery. The larger leaves that the plant produces in its second year of growth were wrapped around fruit to keep it fresh and the tall stems of mullein used to be dried and burned as tapers in funeral processions and at other times to give light as well.

Other uses including medicinal

In addition to being a useful domestic commodity, great mullein was a useful and valuable medical herb. It was beneficial in the treatment of scorpion stings, eye complaints, toothache, tonsillitis and coughs. The leaves were dried and made into

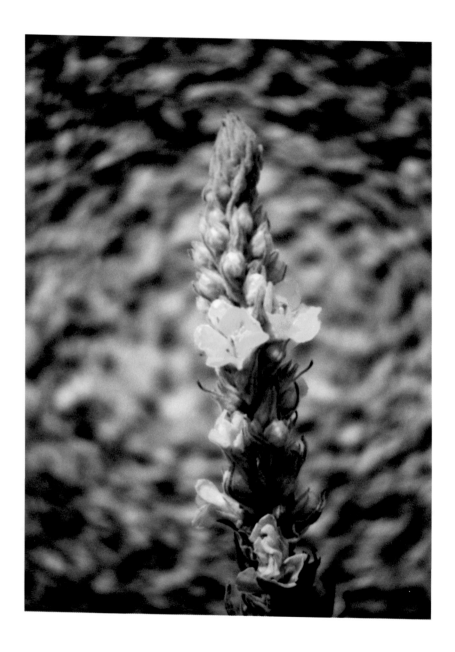

Great Mullein

herbal tobacco and smoked to give relief from asthma and tuberculosis. The flowers could also be infused and made into an oil, which proved helpful in treating haemorrhoids and ear infections.

Poachers found the seeds of the plant very useful too. They discovered that if the seeds were thrown into a pond they stupefied the fish, which could then be lifted out by hand.

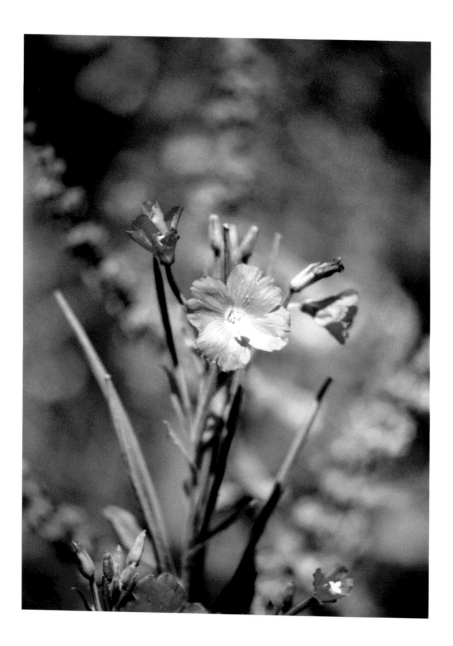

Great Willowherb

Great Willowherb
Llysiau'r Milwr
Epilobium hirsutum

Description

Confusingly, this is not the largest of the willowherbs, a distinction which belongs to the rosebay willowherb. It is, however, tall, with bright pink or purple flowers about 25mm across. These have four petals, notched in the centre, and grow individually on short stalks on the upper part of the stem. The flowers appear through most of the summer, and give rise to long thin seed pods which ultimately split and release feathery airborne seeds. The leaves are long, slender and pointed, usually growing in opposite pairs. Great willowherb usually grows in profusion in damp places.

Naming History

This tall, softly hairy plant is sometimes called 'great hairy willowherb', to tell it apart from the smaller non-hairy species. In fact the specific name *hirsutum* also means 'hairy'. Lyte, the sixteenth century botanist, was born around 1529. He made an English translation of Dodoen's herbal, published in 1578 under the title of *A niewe herbal, or historie of plantes*. In his version he used the name 'willowherb', to describe this group of plants, because of the similarity in the shape of the leaves to that of the willow.

The sixteenth-century Lancastrian botanist Thomas Penny recorded yet another name. *Epilobium hirsutum* was also known as the 'milner flower', or the 'miller's flower', because it looked so pretty growing in abundance beside the mills.

Folklore

Another very attractive country name for this plant is 'codlins and cream'. It may have been given this name because when the leaves are bruised, they smell like boiled apples. Great willowherb was originally given the name of 'codlins and cream' by John Gerard in his *Herbal* which he wrote in 1597. Here he describes it as 'codded willow herbe', because the "flower groweth at the top of the stalke, coming out of the end of a small long codde". So the name 'codlin willow-herb', almost certainly came from 'codded willow herb', the willow-herb of the codlin or cooking apple. Codlins were often boiled in milk and then eaten with cream. This resembled the rosy petals and creamy-white stigmas of the flowers.

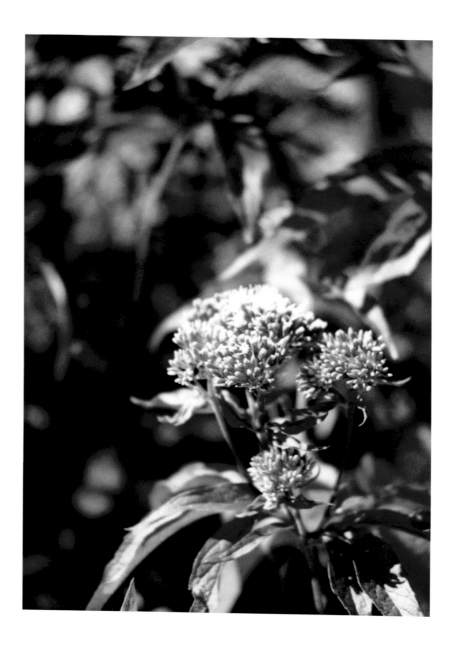

Hemp Agrimony

Hemp Agrimony
Y Byddon Chwerw
Eupatorium cannabinum

Description

This is a tall, sturdy, but surprisingly inconspicuous plant. The reddish stems carry clusters of pointed, toothed leaves at intervals, at which points the stem tends to branch as well. The composite flowers are made up of of tight clusters of pinkish-mauve florets, forming rather flat-topped heads, and can be seen from July to September.

Habitat

Hemp agrimony tends to occur in patches, mostly in damp areas in woods and hedgerows, and on waste ground and marshy places, and is generally seen in company with other tall species, which reduces the chance of casual observation.

Naming History

This plant used to be classified along with tall, yellow-spiked agrimony, and it got its common name from its hemp-like leaves. This is reiterated in the specific name *cannabinum* which is from the same root as the name *cannabis* for the Indian hemp (*Cannabis sativa*) due to their superficial resemblance.

The generic name *Eupatorium* is after Mithridates VI Eupator, King of Pontus and Bithynia (c120 BC to c63 BC). A man of parts, he had received a Greek education, spoke 22 languages and made a great collection of pictures and statues. Among his interests was toxicology, the study of poisons, and he is reputed to have made himself immune from assassination by means of an antidote of his own devising. It is supposed to have contained 46 or more ingredients, one of the chief of which was hemp agrimony... Should you fear assassination yourself, you may care to try this, but no guarantee is given.

Other uses including medicinal

The medical properties of hemp agrimony are many and varied, so maybe Mithridates had some knowledge after all. Long ago it was used as a gentle laxative and for treating eye rheum (sticky eye), in fact the Greeks thought it would be beneficial in treating cataracts. It was also said to be a useful diuretic, and the leaves, boiled and made into an infusion, were said to relieve chest complaints such as catarrh, influenza, coughs and colds, and even arthritis and rheumatism. During the Middle Ages it was widely used as a wound herb and was also thought to be good in the helping of problem skin and scurvy. The Anglo-Saxons even thought that it warded off the Devil.

Modern research has revealed that this plant may also have immune-boosting properties, which could prove useful in treating colds and fevers and may possibly prove beneficial in the treatment of AIDS.

Herb Bennet, Wood Avens
Llysiau f'Anwylyd
Geum urbanum L.

Description

Herb bennet is a medium to tall, very slender plant. The leaves are widely spaced and oval, with lobes near the base, tending to grow at stem junctions. The small yellow flowers can be seen from May to September, and are about 10mm across, five-petalled, with small green sepals visible between the petals. In the autumn these give rise to small hooked fruits, designed to catch in animals' fur for seed dispersal.

Habitat

Herb bennet is commonly found in woods and shady places where the soil is rich.

Naming History

The name herb bennet is not of English origin. It was known and revered in mediaeval France for its powers over the spirits of darkness, and was called, in Latin, the 'blessed herb', *Herba Benedicta*. Since the mediaeval French peasants were often not all that fluent in Latin, the name came to be associated with Saint Benoit.

Folklore

When they are dug up, the roots smell like cloves, and in the Middle Ages the fragrance was thought to repel evil. It was said that if the root was kept in one's house, the Devil would be rendered powerless and flee from the scent. Hence the herb was considered to be blessed above all other herbs.

Other uses including medicinal

In the sixteenth century, herb bennet was grown in gardens as a pot herb. Gerard called it "the common garden Avens", and it was used as a medical herb. It was boiled in pottage or broth or decocted in wine against an upset stomach, wind, stitch, and "the biting of venomous beasts". In practical terms, the scent of the root repels moths as well as the Devil, and Gerard recommends their use: "The rootes taken up in autumn and dried, do keep garments from being eaten with Mothes, and make them to have an excellent good odour".

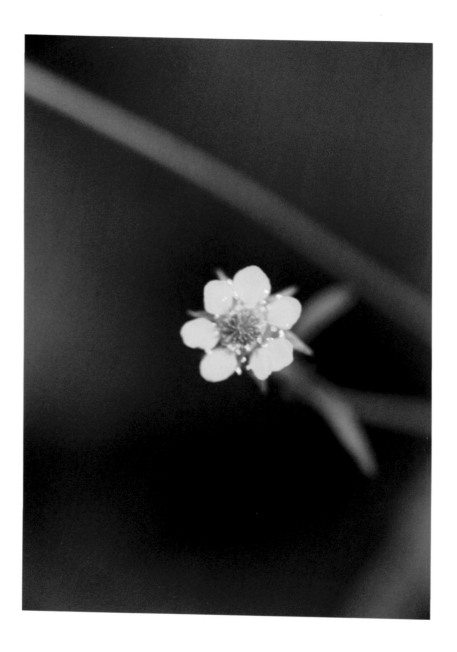

Herb Bennet, Wood Avens

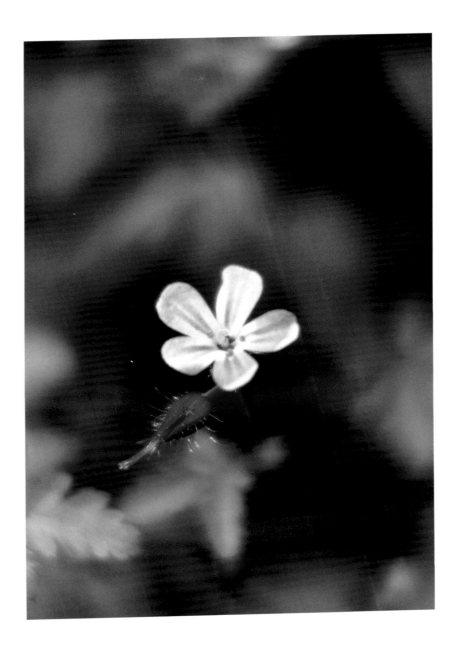

Herb Robert

Herb Robert
Llysiau'r Llwynog, Dail Robin
Geranium robertianum

Description

This common but rather inconspicuous plant grows fairly low to the ground, with three-lobed, deeply-cut leaves, which are initially green but frequently redden later. The flowers grow in small groups at the top of the stem, and are about 20mm across with five pinkish-purple petals. These can be seen from April to November, and give rise to the characteristic fruit, bulbous at the base with a long thin protrusion, somewhat resembling the head and bill of a crane and giving rise to the family name of cranesbills.

Habitat

Herb Robert prefers shady places, and is frequently found in woodlands and woodland margins, sometimes on rocks and shingle.

Naming History

Nobody really knows why 'Robert' was used in the common and specific names of this attractive little flower. It could be after St Robert who was the founder of the Cistercian Order. His day is commemorated on the 29th April, around the time when this little plant is coming into flower. Another and probably the most likely suggestion is that it comes from the Latin word *rubor*, meaning red on account of the colour of the flowers. Geranium comes from the Greek *geranos*, meaning 'crane', (the bird, not the machine), on account of the long seed body resembling a crane's bill. Indeed other members of this family are all called cranesbills.

Folklore

It has even been suggested that the name 'Robert' is a corruption of an older name 'rubwort', and that it could even commemorate the virtues of Robin Hood! Long ago country people thought that Robin Hood was originally an elf who turned into an outlaw, and was linked with the mischievous Robin Goodfellow, who haunted both houses and woodland. This could be related to the plant's colour, hairiness and the candlestick-shaped fruit. Indeed sixteenth century descriptions of Robin Goodfellow make him out to be a hairy goblin, wearing a red suit and having a ruddy complexion. He usually carries a candle-stick and is often associated with 'Kit' and the candlestick, or Jack-o-Lantern, the grotesque face carved in a pumpkin and illuminated at Halloween.

Other uses including medicinal

Despite its rather sinister associations, herb Robert was a very useful medical herb. It was often used as an eye lotion and as a mouthwash for sore throats and mouth ulcers, and still is today. It was recognised as a wound herb and even considered to be able to mend fractures, it was also used to treat milk retention. Culpeper described it as a herb of Venus and commended its use against 'the stone' and to stop bleeding. "It speedily heals wounds and is effectual in old ulcers in the privy parts or elsewhere. A decoction of it has been of service in obstructions of the kidneys and in gravel."

For modern use, the crushed leaves of herb Robert are still used as a compress for healing wounds. The dried herb can also be made into an infusion with boiling water, and taken to treat peptic ulcer, simple diarrhoea and internal haemorrhage. This infusion is also suitable for diabetics as it lowers blood sugar levels, and the freshly crushed leaves rubbed on the arms and legs make an excel-lent mosquito repellent. I have tried this for myself, and it works!

The Scottish discovered another use for the plant in the treatment of cancer. An infusion was made by dicing the whole plant and then adding the pieces to boiling water for an hour. They also believed it was an effective remedy for skin cancer. In fact even as late as the 1920s it was still being prescribed by a herbal-ist in the Lochend district of Invernesshire, who claimed to have cured several people with it. The Gaelic name of 'lus-an-eallain' (cancer weed) reflects this popular usage.

In Pen-Caer in Pembrokeshire, herb Robert was used to treat 'red water' or 'ddwr coch', (blood in the urine) in cattle. It was mixed with buttermilk and fed to the cows.

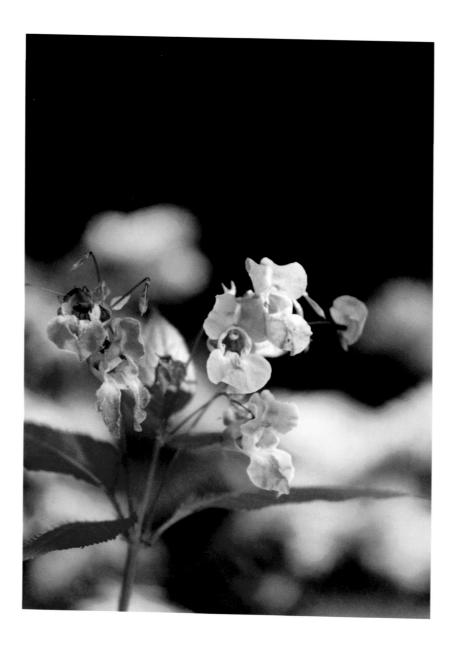

Himalayan Balsam

Himalayan Balsam
Jac y Neidiwr
Impatiens glandulifera

Description

This magnificent plant can sometimes grow up to five feet in height or more. It has a thick, often reddish, hollow stem, which can be anything up to one or two inches in diameter. The large, dark green, lanceolate leaves can reach up to fifteen inches in length. These are stalked, toothed along the edge, and grow opposite each other, or in threes up the stem.

The flowers are large and lipped, the curved petals forming a hollow enclosure with the nectaries at the base designed to attract insects inside, and bear a resemblance to a policeman's helmet, hence the country name. They vary from very pale to dark pink and grow in clusters on long stems at the end of the stalk. In late summer, these give way to long seed pods with a trigger hair on the end. When touched, this causes the ripe pod to split down two lines, and each side curls back on itself. This happens very fast and the seeds are hurled away for several feet by the movement.

Habitat

Himalayan balsam grows prolifically in almost any open space, especially by streams, and competes successfully with many native flowers.

Naming History

The word balsam comes, via Latin and Greek, from the Hebrew word *basam* meaning spice, and was applied to anything fragrant, healing, or yielding aromatic oil. The Himalayan balsam belongs to a group of plants which have some of these properties. The name Himalayan, comes, prosaically enough, from the area in which the plant was first found. A British colloquial name is 'policeman's helmet' from the shape of the flowers. 'Oriental jewelweed' comes from America, possibly from the colourful appearance of a large bank of the plant in flower.

Folklore

Himalayan balsam was introduced into this country from the Himalayas in 1839. It was originally cultivated as a greenhouse annual by gardeners who never imagined the career ahead of it or what a pest it was destined to become. It was planted in borders and grew well, but it had escaped to stream banks by 1855. Now, after nearly 150 years, it grows prolifically and its pink to purple flowers can be seen on nearly every river bank and stream. This plant is extremely successful and spreads everywhere, so it is unwise to plant it in your garden. It is great fun to touch the seed capsules which snap open throwing the seeds a considerable distance. This pastime is very tempting, which all helps to add to this plant's success, and prompted Erasmus Darwin (1731-1802), grandfather of Charles Darwin, to write these following lines:

> With fierce distracted eye Impatiens stands,
> Swells her pale cheeks and brandishes her hands,
> With rage and hate the astonished groves alarms
> And hurls her infants from her frantic arms.

Other uses including medicinal

Himalayan Balsam is used in some modern commercial herbal remedies, to combat irritability and nervous tension.

The young leaves and shoots are edible when cooked. The high mineral content, particularly calcium oxalate, can be harmful if the plant is eaten raw, but cooking or drying will destroy this. The plant can, however, be injurious to people who suffer from rheumatism, gout or arthritis, or anyone who cannot tolerate high acidity in the diet.

The seeds can be eaten raw, should you care to run the risk of being shot by exploding pods while collecting them, and are said to have a pleasing nutty flavour. They also yield an edible oil (hence the 'balsam' nomenclature) which can (if obtained in sufficient quantity – risk of getting shot again) be used for lighting.

Hogweed
Efwr, Pannas y Fuwch
Heracleum sphondylium

Description

Hogweed is a tall, strong, self-supporting plant. It belongs to a family of flowers known as the umbellifers, so called because the flowers consist of a number of florets on stems arranged like the ribs of an umbrella. These florets are pink or white and may be seen at any time from May to November. The giant hogweed (*Heracleum mantegazzianum*), illustrated here, is even taller and may grow higher than a man. The leaves are large and deeply indented on both edges.

Habitat

Both hogweed and giant hogweed are common and widespread, being found especially in grassy places, hedgerows and woodland margins.

Naming History

Hogweed is also known as 'cow parsnip', probably because both common names mean that the root is not fit for human consumption, but can be fed to cows and pigs. In fact cow parsnip is a book name invented by William Turner (1548): "It may be called in Englishe Cow-persnepe or rough Persnepe". It is also a direct translation from the Welsh 'pannas' meaning 'parsnip' and 'fuwch' meaning 'cow'. However, the generic name *Heracleum* is after the Greek hero Heracles (Hercules) because of its giant size and getting it out of your garden is like the labours of Heracles. The specific name *sphondylium* comes from the Italian *'spondilo'*, which originally derives from the Greek word meaning *'vertebra'*, probably because of the hollow internodes on the stems.

Other uses including medicinal

Hogweed was used all over the country as pig fodder, and villagers used to pick bundles of this free harvest from the hedgerows for the sties. The sprouting leaves and shoots are said to taste rather like asparagus, so perhaps the pigs had a discerning appetite. This can be illustrated by some of the old local country names, which include 'swineweed' and 'pig's food' from Devon, 'humpy-scrumples' and in Odhran, Ireland, 'pig's bubble'.

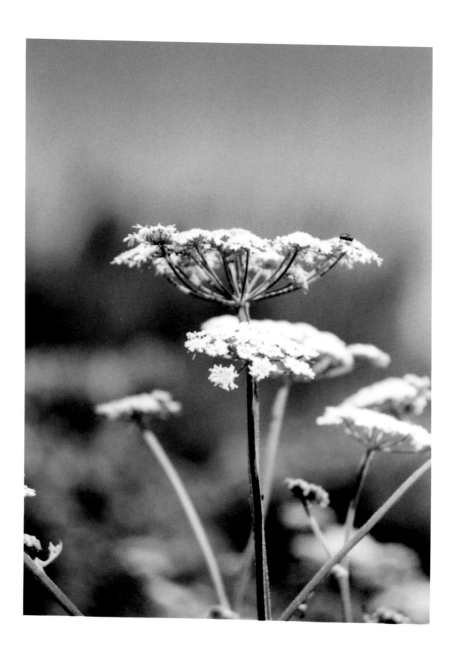

Hogweed

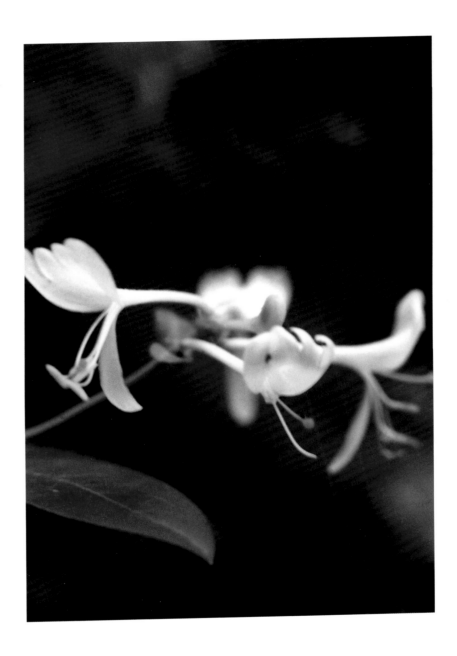

Honeysuckle

Honeysuckle
Gwyddfid, Llaeth y Gaseg
Lonicera periclymenum

Description

Honeysuckle is a climbing plant, supporting itself on the stems of nearby trees and shrubs by the use of twisting tendrils. Unlike many climbers, though, it is a woody plant, and the stems harden into the shape which they adopt as the plant grows. The pale green leaves grow in opposite pairs at intervals on the stem, and appear surprisingly early, being visible from mid-winter onwards. The distinctive cream to dark pink flowers can be seen from June to October, and consist of a number of tubular two-lipped florets around a central point. The flower is quite heavily scented and attracts those insects, such as butterflies, which have a long proboscis able to reach the nectaries at the bottom of the tubes.

Habitat

Honeysuckle is occasionally seen in mature hedges, but more often can be found in the depths of woodland where there is plenty of support for climbers.

Naming History

Honeysuckle is so named from the old idea that bees extracted honey from it, but in fact it is entirely useless to the bee which does not have a long proboscis. However there was a belief that if the juice from a honeysuckle leaf was squeezed and then spread around a bee hive, this would keep the bees happy and make then stay for a long time.

Some attractive country names include 'woodbine', presumably because of the way honeysuckle entwines itself around saplings, 'gramophone horns', and 'lamps of scent' both from Somerset. 'Lady's fingers' from Yorkshire, Dorset and Northumberland relate to the long, slender trumpets described by William Bullein, in his *Book of Simples* (1562): "...wyth his long winding stalkes, and tender leaves, opening or spreding forth his sweete Lillies, like ladies fingers, emong the thorns or bushes".

Folklore

Farmers were opposed to picking honeysuckle because they thought it would give them an unsuccessful second crop of hay, although honeysuckle was beneficial to them as well. It was one of the flowers used in May Day celebrations to drive away evil, and was especially effective in protecting cows, milk and butter. This belief was particularly common in the Highlands of Scotland.

Because of the way it entwines itself around other plants, like a tight embrace, honeysuckle is often associated with love. In fact in the *Language of Flowers*, fidelity and affection are symbolised by the honeysuckle, and in some areas it is even called 'hold me tight'. Because of its heady fragrance it was once believed that the smell of it engendered amorous thoughts, so it was therefore considered unwise to bring it indoors into the presence of young girls. It might give them the wrong ideas! However if an older and more mature person picked it, then the fragrance would give them dreams of love and matrimony. A classical reference to the honeysuckle can be found in the 'Song of Solomon':

> I am the rose of Sharon,
> and the lily of the valleys.
> As the lily among thorns,
> so is my love among the daughters.

The 'lily among thorns' is often equated with this flower.

Under the name of woodbine, honeysuckle also has a more sinister use. A twining and constricting plant, it could be used by a suitably qualified witch or warlock to bind or constrain the actions of an enemy. In the ballad 'Willie's Lady', the witch used various means of preventing the birth of the lady's child, including planting a 'bush o' woodbine' before the lady's bower. Unfortunately for the witch, her schemes were frustrated by the house goblin who told Willie how to remove the spells. Once the constricting honeysuckle was overcome, the child could make a safe entry into the world.

Other uses including medicinal

The medical uses of honeysuckle are many and various. Culpeper described a decoction of the leaves as being a remedy for a sore throat or a cough and "to open obstructions of the liver and spleen".

Nowadays honeysuckle can be used as a laxative, expectorant, diuretic, diaphoretic and emetic. It also contains natural antibiotics and salicylic acid from which aspirin is obtained.

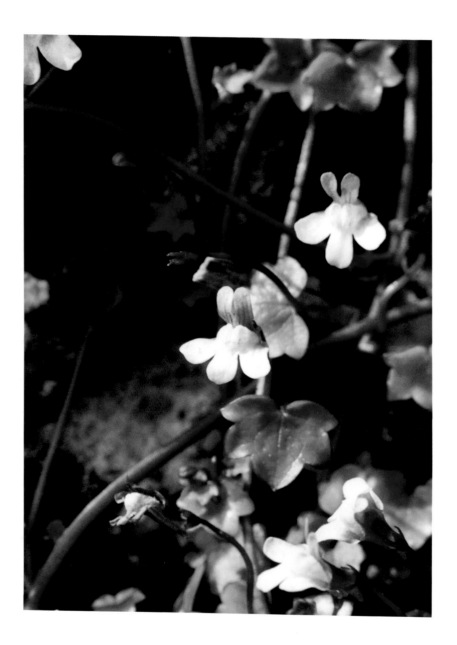

Ivy-Leaved Toadflax

Ivy-Leaved Toadflax
Trwyn y Llo Dail Iorwg, Llin y Fagwyr
Cymbalaria muralis

Description

This is a small, trailing perennial plant, with, as its name suggests, ivy-shaped leaves, growing on long stalks. The flowers, which may be seen from April to November, are small, no more than 10mm across, purple in colour with a central yellow spot, and are heavily lobed with the main petals at the bottom.

Habitat

Ivy-leaved toadflax is originally adapted for life on rock faces and is particularly adept at distributing its seeds to appropriate locations. Each seed grows on the tip of a slender stalk, and when the seed is ripe, the stalk grows in a twisting fashion, rather like a tendril, until the seed on the end becomes caught in a crack in the rock or stone wall. The seed, snugly ensconced, becomes detached, germinates, and a new plant grows in a still more inaccessible position than its parent. Thus this plant can be found growing on vertical stone faces that are denied to other flowers, particularly ruined castles.

Naming History

The distinctive ivy-shaped leaves give the plant its common name of 'ivy-leaved toadflax'. The generic name *Cymbalaria* is from the Greek *Kymbalon* meaning 'symbol' and refers to the shape of the leaves in some species, whereas the specific name *muralis* simply means that it grows on walls. The Welsh name 'Trwyn y llo dail iorwg' means 'ivy-leaved calf's nose', with 'calf's nose' presumably referring to the shape of the flower, the two yellow blotches representing eyes and the three lobes the mouth and nose. This is further enhanced by the Hertfordshire name of 'nanny goats' mouths'.

Folklore

Ivy-leaved toadflax was originally introduced into this country as a garden plant early in the seventeenth century. William Coys, a well known amateur gardener, planted it in his garden at North Ockenden in Essex. By 1640, ivy-leaved toadflax had become very popular and was a familiar sight in gardens and must have made many separate escapes.

By 1724 it was growing on the walls surrounding the Chelsea Physic Garden and the Botanic Garden in Oxford. In fact over the span of the last three centuries, this attractive plant has spread onto most of the walls, castles and old ruins around Great Britain. At one time botanists used to debate whether or not the plant was a native to the country. About 150 years ago, while on holiday in Wales, a botanist noticed the plant growing on a rock near Barmouth, and reckoned it was too far from the houses to have escaped from a garden. He reported his discovery to *Loudon's Magazine of Natural History* and received this answer from a correspondent: "I here declare that several years ago, in one of my numerous tours through that [Barmouth] and other mountainous regions, I carried a box of seeds of this beautiful and tenacious plant which I distributed in appropriate places on rocks, ruins, churches, castles and bridges where I have since beheld it thriving in tresses and festoons to my fullest satisfaction. I particularly remember sowing it on the rock he mentions." Ever since, this wall-loving plant has continued spreading its domain over our ancient buildings and has staked its claim as a plant belonging to Britain.

Kingcup (Marsh Marigold, Mayblobs)
Melyn y Gors, Gold y Gors
Caltha palustris

Description

Kingcup leaves are large, glossy and horseshoe shaped. They have a bluntly serrated edge, are often paler and mottled on the upper surface, and appear shortly before the flowers. The buttercup-like flowers are large and showy. They are a shining golden yellow and measure up to 50mm across. They can be either solitary or in bunches of two or three on the stem.

Habitat

Kingcups can be found growing in marshes and other wet places, usually in shallow water. Their shining, sun-like flowers open while the year is still colourless and cold and last into May. They help to brighten up damp areas such as grey moors and wet meadows, or the black mud by the roots of alder trees.

Naming History

The common name 'kingcup' almost certainly means a large, kingsized buttercup-like flower, although it is possible that it could have come from the Anglo-Saxon word 'copp', meaning 'head', and it is said that the unopened flower bud resembles the gold studs that were worn by kings. The Anglo-Saxons also thought the tight flower buds looked rather like galls, and gave them the name of 'meargealla' or 'horse-gall', which later became changed to 'marigold'. The name 'Mayblobs' meaning 'mere', 'marsh', and 'blob' or 'bleb', meaning 'bladder', could well be of Anglo-Saxon origin too, in reference to the unopened flower buds, although it is far more likely to be because they are still in flower during the month of May.

The generic name *Caltha* is from the Greek *kalathos*, 'goblet', again on account of the flower's shape and the specific name *palustris*, simply means that it grows in marshes.

Folklore

It always used to be considered unlucky to bring kingcups into the house before the first of May, although in Shropshire, particularly in Edgmond, on May Day, every householder decorated their houses with a bunch of marigolds, arranged

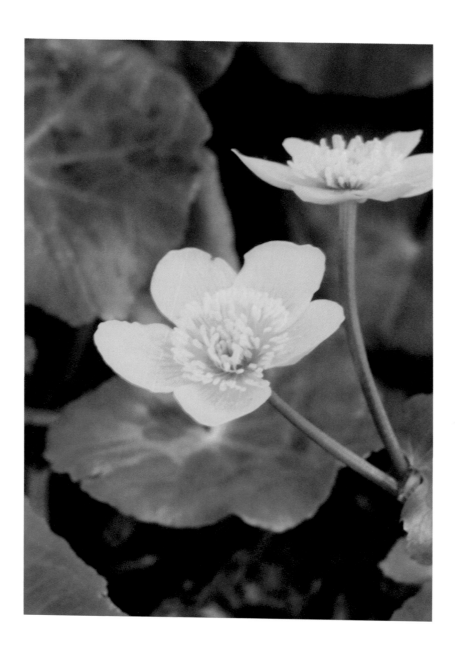

Kingcup (*Marsh Marigold, Mayblobs*)

stalks upward, until as late as 1876. But after the calendar changed in 1752 the traditional may flower was not yet in bloom, so the marsh marigold had to take its place. This seems to have been a continuation of a belief that the flowers would offer protection against lightning in the thunder storms of early summer. An Irish superstition went further, bunches of kingcups hung over the doors of a cowshed would ward off witches and fairies and ensure the fertility of the cattle. They even went so far as to entwine kingcups into a hoop with rowan blossoms, from which they suspended two balls, one covered in gold paper and the other with silver, which were intended to represent the sun and the moon. This may have been a further expression of a fertility rite, but latterly seems to have been a traditional decoration for May Day festivities.

An elderly gentleman recalls from his childhood memories, that it was once a tradition in his Shropshire village to gather kingcups or may flowers from his local meadow on the eve of the thirtieth of April. Before nightfall he would put a kingcup through the letterbox of every house in the village. This was to make sure that evil fairies did not enter the houses before May Day. The older residents were particularly superstitious and would remind him not to forget them.

Other uses including medicinal

The burning juice from the stems of this plant used to be applied to warts.

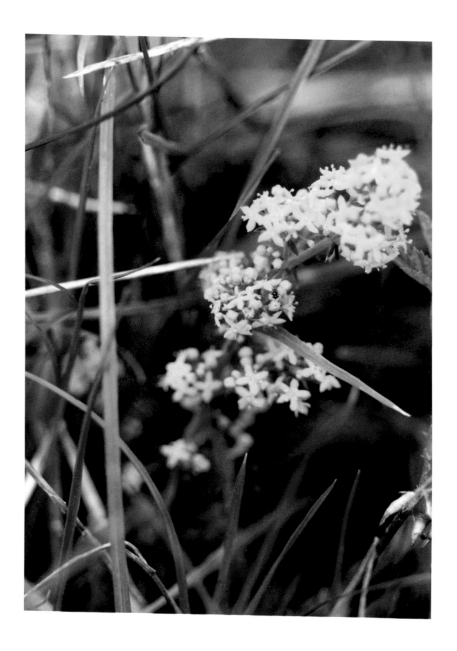

Lady's Bedstraw

Lady's Bedstraw
Llysiau'r Cywer, Briwydden Felen
Galium verum

Description

Lady's bedstraw is a low sprawling plant, with narrow, dark green leaves growing in whorls of about ten at intervals up the stem. The flowers are small, bright yellow and grow in clusters at the top of the stems, appearing from June to September.

Habitat

Lady's bedstraw is commonly found in dry grassy places, such as open hillsides and established sand dunes. Being a low-growing plant, it is not found in fields where the grass grows tall or where there is considerable shade.

Naming History

The common name of lady's bedstraw derives from the legend related below. The element 'straw' is the same word as the verb 'to strew' meaning to lay or scatter, and does not refer to dried grass stems.

Folklore

A mediaeval legend from northern Europe stated that during the nativity Mary lay on a bed of lady's bedstraw and bracken. The bracken refused to acknowledge the child, thereby losing its flowers. The lady's bedstraw however welcomed the child and burst into bloom, to find that as a reward its flowers had changed from white to gold. Mary is said to have put some lady's bedstraw into Jesus's manger and this was the only plant that the donkey did not eat. During the evening or when the air is damp, the flowers of lady's bedstraw smell like honey, but when they dry out they smell like hay. This fragrance made it pleasant for use in bedding, in the days when a mattress consisted of dried vegetation, and presumably the same held good two thousand years ago. In addition to this, wealthy ladies used to stuff their pillows with this herb, because it was a flea repellent, and the pleasant fragrance helped to promote sleep.

Central European superstitions took this a little further. Women who were about to give birth put lady's bedstraw in their beds because they believed it would make the birth easier and safer. Women who had recently given birth, considered themselves vulnerable to attack from demons and infections, so they would not enter another house unless they had some lady's bedstraw in their shoes.

Other uses including medicinal

In northern parts of the country, lady's bedstraw was used to give the yellow colour to cheese, and the plant was also a useful substitute to rennet. In Gloucestershire nettle juice was added to give the distinctive flavour to Double Gloucester cheese, although this method was getting rare towards the end of the eighteenth century. This can be further illustrated by some of the local country names of 'cheese rennet', from Shropshire, 'cheese-running', from Ireland and 'rennet', from northern England.

Lesser Celandine
Llygad Ebrill
Ranunculus ficaria

Description

Lesser celandine is a low hairless perennial with rather fleshy, dark green, heart-shaped leaves which appear before the flowers. The flowers themselves are bright yellow, usually consisting of eight to twelve narrow pointed petals, with a ring of stamens in the centre. They appear in the early spring, around March, and flower through to May.

Habitat

This yellow flower, which superficially resembles a buttercup, can be seen glinting in fields and hedges in March, heralding the coming of spring. It will grow on most soil types but prefers rich pastureland.

Naming History

Lesser celandine is sometimes called 'smallwort', because of the size of the plant, and the common name 'celandine' is of Greek origin. The specific name *ficaria* comes from the small fig-like tubers of the plant's roots. An alternative name, from its ancient medicinal use, is 'pilewort' (see below).

Folklore

The name 'celandine' comes from the Greek word *chelicon* meaning 'swallow', perhaps because the plant is in flower when the swallows arrive, perhaps because the Roman historian Pliny believed that lesser celandine was used by swallows to improve their nestlings' eyesight. The fig-like roots were also popularly believed to resemble a cow's udders because of the way they are arranged, and the yellow petals signified butter. In the Scottish Highlands farmers hung a bunch of tubers on the cowshed, or on the cow's fetters, to increase the yield of cream in the cow's milk.

The nineteenth-century poet William Wordsworth was particularly fond of lesser celandines, and was inspired to write these words about them:

> There is a flower that shall be mine,
> Tis the little celandine.

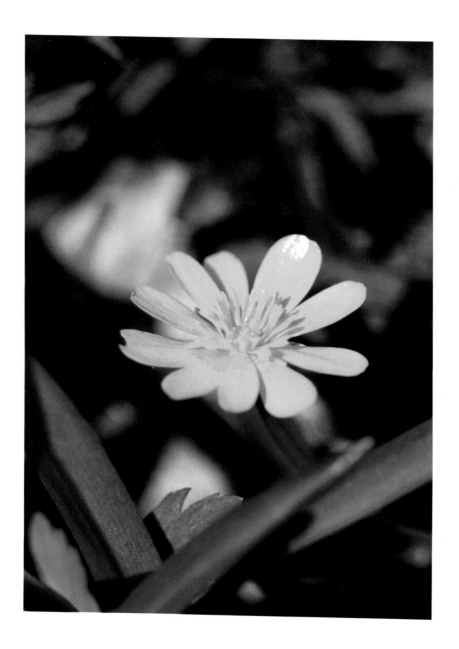

Lesser Celandine

Other uses including medicinal

Culpeper describes how an infusion of the leaves and root "doth wonderfully help piles and haemorrhoids, also kernals by the ears and throat, called the 'King's Evil'".

A local Welsh name for lesser celandine is 'ddail peils' or 'pile leaves'. The early Welsh apothecaries discovered their healing properties for treating piles, and this is likely to have been one of the remedies formalised and handed down by the Physicians of Myddfai. The physical appearance of the roots, with bumps and nodules, reminded them of the appearance of piles, and on the principle of 'Athrawiaeth y Arwyddnodau' ('Teaching of the Tokens [signs]'), attributed healing powers of the one to be used on the other. This principle was common in early medicine, where if the appearance of an affliction was mimicked by something in nature, it was believed that that would be a cure for the affliction. Therefore a simple concoction was made by crushing the leaves and roots of the plant and boiling them in non-salted buttermilk. This was then applied to the afflicted area. It also proved to be beneficial in the treatment of swollen glands, behind the ears and in the throat. The Welsh made a poultice to ease swelling, to treat boils and carbuncles:

1) Collect fennel, garlic and celandine
2) Crush fine 1lb of the mix
3) Add vinegar and non salted butter
4) Make into poultice and leave for a while then place on afflicted area

Lesser celandine is still used for the treatment of haemorrhoids today. It can be used as an ointment or drunk as an infusion. Because of its bright yellow colour it was also considered to be useful in the treatment of jaundice, and the juice from the crushed stems was used for 'defaid oddi ar ddwylo' ('taking the sheep off the hands'), or in other words getting rid of warts! Dandelion juice was also used for this purpose.

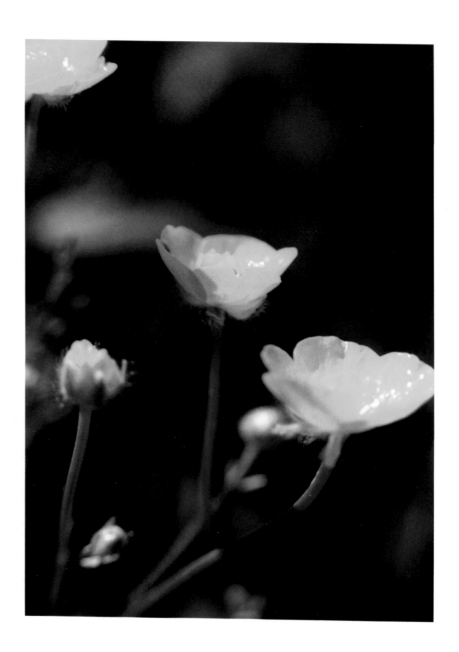

Meadow Buttercup

Meadow Buttercup
Blodyn Melyn, Blodyn Ymenyn
Ranunculus acris

Description

Often found growing amongst long grass, meadow buttercup is a medium tall perennial, with characteristic deeply cut leaves, quite unlike those of bulbous or creeping buttercup. The five-petalled yellow flowers measure about 2-3cm across, with the sepals pressed close to the base of the flower. They appear during April and are in bloom right through to about October.

Habitat

Meadow buttercup, as its name implies, is usually found growing in meadows, roadside verges and damp grassy places.

Naming History

The suffix 'cup' almost certainly refers to the yellow cup-like flower, but it may go back as far as the Anglo-Saxon word 'cop' meaning 'head'. The name buttercup does not seem to have come into everyday use until the middle of the eighteenth century. The Elizabethan botanist John Gerard referred to meadow buttercup as 'butterflower', along with 'kingcob', 'gold knobs' and 'crowfoot', although crowfoot was the name most used by the early botanists. Nowadays every child is taught in the village school that a buttercup is a butter-cup, but this has not destroyed some of the other country names such as 'bache-lor's buttons', 'butter-and-cheese' and 'butter-daisy', or the belief that if you hold a buttercup under your chin, it reflects a yellow glow to show that you like butter. This method was used for divining the truth. Questions would be asked pertaining to fidelity, love and friendship. The yellow glow signified that the person was telling the truth.

The scientific name *Ranunculus* actually comes from the Latin name 'rana' meaning 'frog' because many species of buttercup grow in moist places where frogs are found. However, there is another charming story which tells of a little boy called Ranunculus who was clad in gold and green. He liked to run through the woods and fields singing all the time with a beautiful clear voice. Eventually he annoyed the wood nymphs and they turned him into a buttercup to restore peace to the fields and forests again.

Folklore

A meadow full of yellow buttercups is a beautiful sight in the summer, so much so that at one time farmers believed that fields full of buttercups meant that their cows would have a higher percentage of cream in their milk that year, enabling them to make better quality butter. However the species name *acris* means that buttercups are sour or bitter. They contain a chemical called protoanemonin, which makes pasture land acrid and causes other plants not to grow. Therefore it was believed that if a cow lay down amongst the buttercups, her udder would be bewitched. Even so farmers would still rub their cows' udders with a bunch of buttercups, believing that this would improve the cows' yield for that year. This proved productive, because the bitter taste left on the udders discouraged the calves from feeding, so they were weaned earlier, thus leaving more milk for making butter.

Meadow Cranesbill
Garanbig y Weirglodd
Geranium pratense

Description

This beautiful member of the cranesbill family has the characteristic long 'crane's bill' shaped seed body. The leaves are cut nearly to the base and they turn an attractive shade of tawny red in the autumn. The flowers, which are a beautiful shade of blue measuring about 25-30mm across, appear during the summer months of June to September. It is locally common and, where found, grows in abundance, for example in northern Wiltshire.

Habitat

This plant grows in patches and adds a wonderful splash of colour to grassy areas and roadside verges during the summer months.

Naming History

The crane's bill connection is further illustrated by the generic name *Geranium*, which is thought to have derived from the Greek *geranos*, which also means 'crane', and the specific name *pratense* means that it grows in meadows.

Meadow cranesbill has some attractive local names too; 'blue basins', 'blue buttons', 'blue warrior' and 'granny's bonnets' from Somerset, and 'gypsy' and 'loving Andrews' from Wiltshire. In his version of *Dodoens*, Henry Lyte translated from the German *Gottesgnade* meaning 'grace of God', a lovely name for so pretty a flower.

Other uses including medicinal

Along with water violet, tormentil, raspberry leaves, witch hazel and marigold flowers, meadow cranesbill can be used to treat Leucorrhoea, a vaginal discharge.

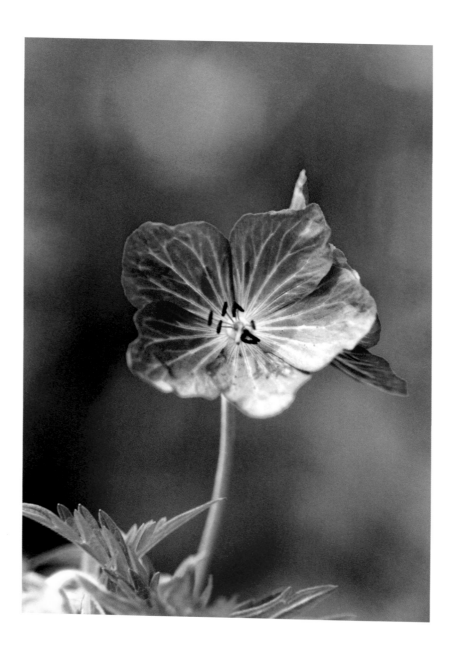

Meadow Cranesbill

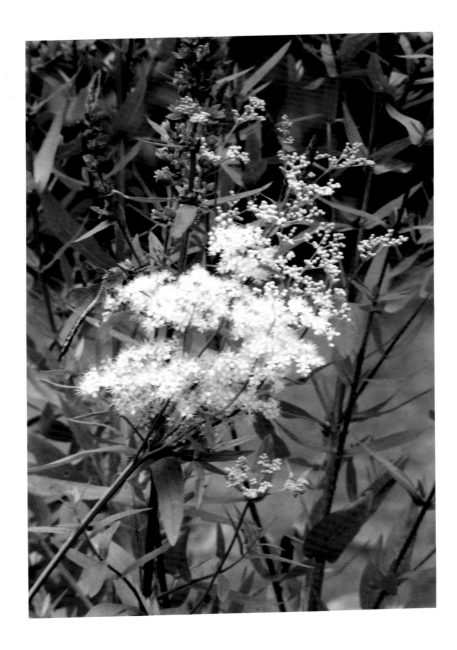

Meadowsweet

Meadowsweet
Erwain, Blodau'r Mel, Llysiau'r Forwyn
Filipendula ulmaria

Description

Meadowsweet is a member of the rose family or Rosaceae. The small, creamy-coloured flowers have five or six petals each, grow in dense clusters, and have a sweet and heady fragrance. The plant grows up to 1.2m (4ft) in height with stiff upright hairless stems and large pinnate leaves on long peduncles.

Habitat

Meadowsweet is also called 'queen of the meadows', as this common perennial can be found growing abundantly in meadows, along roadside verges and in hedges, on the banks of streams and even around the edges of ponds. It flowers throughout the summer from the months of June to September.

Naming History

The name meadowsweet could have come from the Anglo-Saxon words 'mede' or 'medo-wyrt', meaning 'mead' or 'honey-herb', because in the days before sugar was used, the flowers were added to drinks, in order to sweeten them. The specific name *ulmaria*, meaning 'elm-like' is due to the characteristically elm-like shape of the leaves.

Folklore

A traditional Irish legend stated that the moon goddess Aine of Knockaine, who was the goddess of crops and of cattle, gave meadowsweet its beautiful smell. Therefore on account of its sweet smell meadowsweet used to be associated with death and it was considered unlucky to bring some into the house. Surprisingly enough even as late as in 1959 people in Worcestershire still believed that the sweet and heady scent would induce a deep sleep from which a person might not waken. But in contrast the Elizabethans liked the sweet scent of Meadowsweet and would strew it around their houses, to perfume the rooms and dull some of the other odours. In fact a quotation from Gerard says: "the leaves and flowers far excelled all other strewing herbs, for to deck up houses, to strew in chambers, halls and banketting houses in the summertime; for the smell made the heart merry, delighted the senses and did not cause headaches, as some other sweet smelling herbs did".

Another remarkable thing about meadowsweet is that the sweet scent becomes sharper when the plant is crushed, this apparently prompted the Shetland name of 'courtship-and-matrimony', as in Rudyard Kipling;

> Pleasant the snaffle of Courtship, improving the manners and carriage.
> But the colt who is wise will abstain from the terrible thorn-bit of Marriage.

The scent of meadowsweet, while sweet, may become nauseating in quantity and, of old, apothecaries called it 'goat's beard', perhaps because of the cloud of sweet-smelling white flowers. These may also have helped to prompt some of the other country names including 'lady of the meadow' from Somerset, 'maids of the meadow' from Cheshire and in Wales it is called 'llysiau'r forwyn' (the virgin's herbs), perhaps because of its sweet smell. The flowers were used as an early air freshener. A large bunch was put in a pitcher and placed on a windowsill. The scent would pervade the whole house and create a fresh environment for the inhabitants.

In the old Welsh legend, meadowsweet was one of the nine flowers used by the wizards Gwydion and Math to create Blodeuwedd. The story comes from the *Mabinogion*, and it is said that Aranrhod put a curse on the young prince Lleu that he should never have a mortal wife. The two wizards felt sorry for him, and created him a beautiful wife out of flowers, of which it is said that meadowsweet was one. Unfortunately Blodeuwedd was unfaithful to her husband. She fell in love with a hunter, and the two of them decided to kill Lleu, but Lleu did not die, like an ordinary person. He turned into an eagle and flew away. Gwydion heard about this and turned Blodeuwedd into an owl, and she is now hated by all other birds.

Other uses including medicinal

In Nottinghamshire and other northern counties, the small flowers used to be picked and dried and made into a herbal tobacco. It was called 'old man's pepper'. 'Old man' is a common tag for the Devil. Many parts of the plant were used as teas to treat different ailments. An infusion made from the freshly picked tops of this plant promoted sweating, whilst a tea made from the leaves was a good treatment for colds and reducing consumption. The Welsh made tea from the flowers to cure flu and cellulitis, ease kidney and bladder pain, calm nerves and promote sleep:

1) Boil ½ ounce of dried flowers in 1 pint of water
2) Place lid on pot and leave to simmer for 10 minutes
3) Drink 1 cup before breakfast every day for a fortnight

It was considered a good wound herb, both inwardly or outwardly applied, and water distilled from the flowers was considered good for inflammation of the eyes.

Since the discovery in modern times that meadowsweet contains methyl salicylate, it has been used as a successful drug against rheumatism. The salicylate in the flowers is an effective anti-toxin meaning that a tea made from the dried flowers behaved similarly to aspirin with the advantage that the stomach lining was not irritated.

Like many common herbs, meadowsweet is rich in vitamin C and some health-conscious people may certainly have used the herb in sandwiches.

Nipplewort
Cartheig
Lapsana communis

Description

Nipplewort is a slender, medium-tall, hairy annual plant, with small, pointed oval leaves. The flowers are small, less than 20mm across and are bright yellow, carried on long slender stems, and are composed of a number of florets.

Habitat

Nipplewort can be found growing in shady, bare and waste places such as woods and roadside verges, and will quite often turn up as a weed in your garden.

Naming History

The common name not unsurprisingly refers back to when this herb was used in early medicine, when it was used to treat sore nipples. According to the Nuremburg physician and botanist, Joachim Camerarius, in his herbal which he wrote in 1588, *Hortus medicus et philosophicus*, the Prussian apothecaries used to call this herb 'papillaris', because they said that "it was good to heale the ulcers of the nipples of a women's breasts". Eventually 'papillaris' was translated into the English name of 'nipplewort'.

Another reason for the name 'nipplewort', is the nipple-like shape of the buds before they open. The generic name also has a medicinal meaning and comes from the Greek *lapazo*, which indicates that this herb was used as a purgative.

Other uses including medicinal

As mentioned above, nipplewort was used to treat sore nipples and to heal ulcers on women's breasts. It was also used as a purgative.

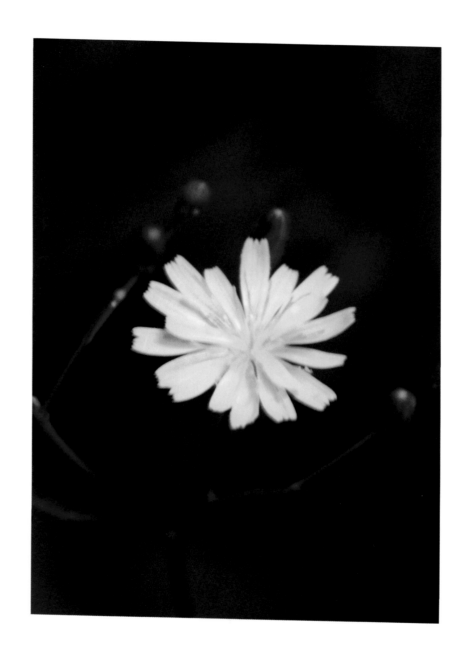

Nipplewort

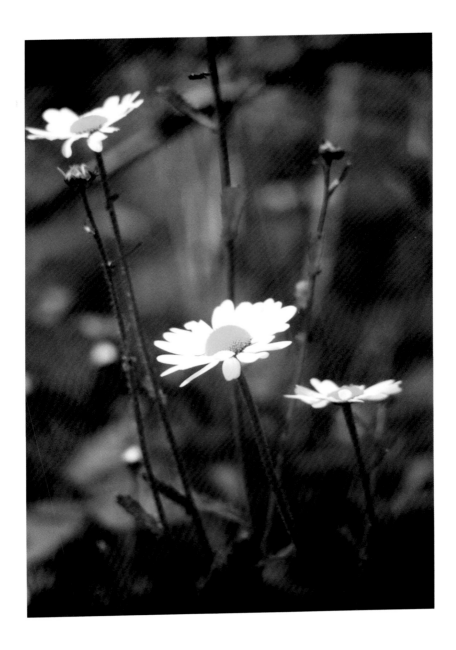

Ox-eye Daisy

Ox-Eye Daisy
Llygad Llo Mawr, Llygad y Dydd Mawr
Chrysanthemum leucanthemum

Description

These magnificent large white daisies flower during the summer months of May to September, with slender deeply-toothed leaves growing upwards and close to the stem. The flowers may be up to 50mm across.

Habitat

Ox-eye daisies are a common sight on waste grassy places and roadside verges.

Naming History

This flower was sometimes called 'moon daisy', because of its white petals and big yellow centre, which gave it the resemblance of the moon or an ox's eye. This is further accentuated by the Greek root of the generic name *crysos* meaning 'gold' and the specific name *leucanthemum* which comes from the Greek *leukos* 'white' refering to the long white ray-like petals. In fact both 'moon daisy' and 'dog daisy' are both old English names. Apparently the name ox-eye daisy did not come into use until the sixteenth century, when perhaps some of the other attractive local names such as 'Billy button' from Lancashire and 'cow's eyes' and 'crazy Bett' from Somerset also started being used.

Folklore

Summer thunderstorms have always been a threat to country folk, damaging, sometimes severely, both dwellings and crops. Before the days of weather forecasts and insurance policies, one precaution against thunder was to hang ox-eye daisies around the doors and across roofs and haylofts, in the belief that this would protect the incumbent against the ravages of lightning. This was particularly so in the Tyrol and parts of Germany, but some Old English names also reflect this superstition, such as thunder daisy and dunder daisy.

Other uses including medicinal

Ox-eye daisy was considered an excellent medical herb too, especially for treatment of breathing problems, such as asthma or consumption. The whole herb, stalks, leaves and flowers were boiled up together, made into a posset and drunk.

It was also thought to be beneficial in the treatment of wounds and ulcers both inwardly or outwardly applied. A decoction of the herb was even said by John Pechey "to cure all diseases that are occasion'd by drinking cold beer when the body is hot". Presumably he meant relieving a wind attack.

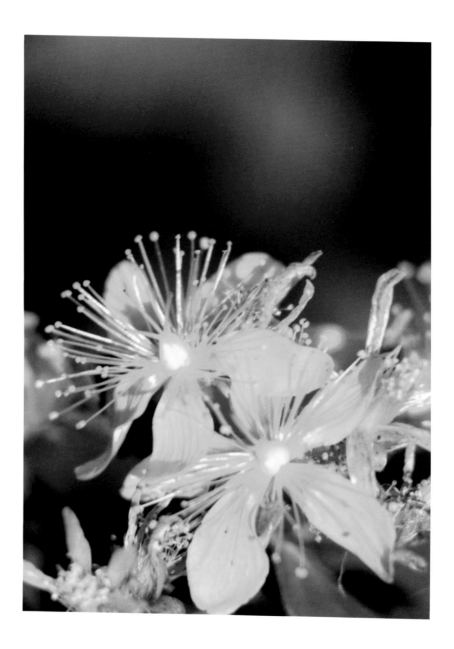

Perforate St John's Wort

Perforate St John's Wort
Dail y Fendigaid, Llysiau Ioan
Hypericum perforatum

Description

This is a medium-sized perennial with five-petalled flowers about 20mm across, and oval pointed leaves growing in pairs. The remarkable thing about the leaves is that they have a number of translucent dots on the surface, and if held up to the light these can clearly be seen. The numerous bright yellow flowers appear between July and September.

Habitat

St John's wort favours grassy and bushy places.

Naming History

It is because the leaves on this plant appear to be covered in tiny holes, that it has the specific name *perforatum* meaning pierced. Long ago it was believed that these holes would ooze blood on 29th August, the date of St John the Baptist's execution. Alternatively another belief states that the holes appear on this day. There are also red spots on the leaves and, when either crushed or bruised, the flowers produce a red juice which supposedly represents St John's blood.

Folklore

A lot of folklore is attached to St John's wort, and country people used to be very superstitious. It was therefore believed that if it was placed in the window on the 24th June, (the day reputed to be the saint's birthday), it would keep away ghosts and witches as well as giving protection against fire and lightning. Its powers were thought to be at their strongest on St John's Eve, so it was ceremoniously gathered while it was still damp with dew. A certain amount of divination came into this also. Unmarried girls believed that if they did this they would be married before the end of the year, and Hertfordshire maidens thought that if they picked a bloom on midsummer night and found it was still fresh in the morning they would very soon be married. Taking this a little further; if a childless woman walked naked to pick it, she would (perhaps not surprisingly) conceive within that year.

Other uses including medicinal

St John's wort is also thought to have taken its name from the Knights of St John of Jerusalem, who used it to treat wounds on the battlefields of the Crusades. On account of its yellow flowers it was thought to be effective against jaundice, and it was used in the treatment of depression and still is today.

A powerful plant, St John's wort need only be used in moderation. Welsh women discovered that the leaves were useful for treating both internal and external bruising and firmly believed that there were none better at lessening pain. A cream created by boiling the leaves in non salty buttermilk was used to reduce swelling.

Pignut
Cneuen Ddaear
Conopodium majus

Description

Pignut belongs to the umbellifer family, meaning that the flowerhead consists of small florets carried on stems arranged like the spokes of an umbrella. The flowers are white, and the whole plant is slender and of medium height. The leaves are slim and feathery.

Habitat

Pignut likes growing in open woods and open grassland such as meadows.

Naming History

The generic name for this plant, *Conopodium*, is descended from the Greek *konos*, 'cone' and *podus* 'foot', probably because the shape of the flowers resembles a foot, with their inwardly turned tips.

Folklore

Pignut was recommended by herbalists as a useful medicine and sometimes for food. In 1694 John Pechey was prompted to write in his *Compleat Herbal of Physical Plants* that "the nuts, peeled and boiled in fresh broth with a little pepper, were very pleasant and nourishing, and better still it was a dish which stimulated venery".

Other uses including medicinal

Pignut has a large tuberous root, which is said to be nut-like in flavour and is eagerly rooted out and eaten by pigs. People enjoyed hunting for these tubers as well, tracing down the white stem and getting their fingers in under the tuber, then scraping the mud off with a pocket knife and eating it with relish, enjoying its crisp substance and clean taste. Unfortunately, the pignut or earthnut, although it was such a good vegetable, could never be cultivated because it would not thrive on tilled land. So it always had to be gathered from the wild.

Pignut was recommended by herbalists as a useful medicine and sometimes for food.

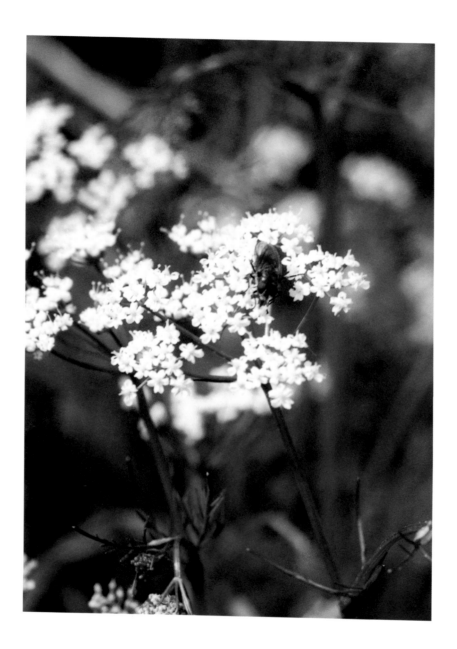

Pignut

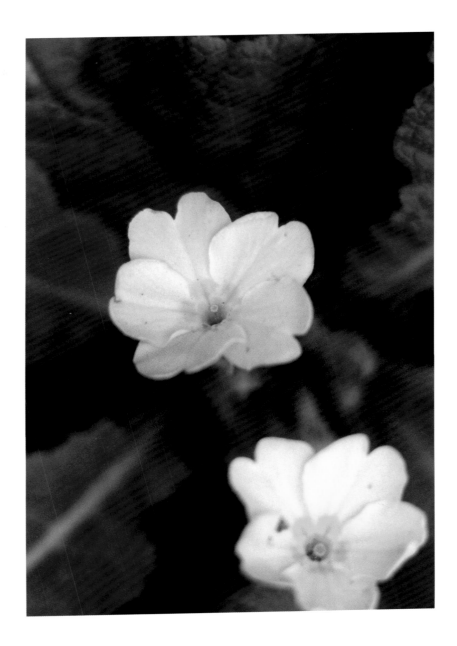

Primrose

Primrose
Briallen, Blodau Llo Bach
Primula vulgaris

Description

This low-growing perennial has dark green, lanceolate leaves with a crinkly surface covered in fine hairs to deter insects. The leaves bear resemblance to those of the cowslips and the rarer oxslips to whom this plant is related. The flowers appear during March and bloom throughout the spring, but may occasionally be seen during a mild winter. These pale yellow, five-petalled flowers grow on long attenuated stalks from the base of the leaves. The flowers are of two varieties; pin-eyed and thrum-eyed depending on the prominance of the stigma. This helps to avoid the problem of self-pollination.

Habitat

The primrose, from the Latin *Prima rosa*, is a familiar sight growing in carpets beside motorways and railway cuttings, grassy verges and woodland banks.

Naming History

The common name of primrose came via the early English name 'primrole' or 'pryme rolles' which descended from the French name *primevere*, which originated from the Latin *primus* 'first' and *ver* 'spring', because it is one of the earliest flowers to appear after the long winter. There may have been some confusion in the translation from the French between 'primevere' and 'primerose', which is in fact French for hollyhock, a tall plant with a much more rose-like flower. The generic name *Primula* shows it is classified in the *Primulaceae* family, and the specific name *vulgaris* means it is commonly found.

Folklore

Perhaps because of the cheerful yellow against the dull colours of the winter countryside, primroses have long been associated with folklore. The brown marks in the centre of primroses are said to be the rust marks left behind by the keys of heaven when St Peter mislaid them, and they were left out all night lying on the primroses.

As a corollary with spring and fertility, they became involved with superstitions about domestic fowl, particularly hens. In east Suffolk and Sussex it was considered unlucky to bring a posy of less than thirteen primroses into the house. Thirteen eggs was considered to be the size of the standard clutch.

It was considered very serious to have just one bloom in the house, because this meant that only one egg would hatch from a day's clutch and, even more serious, it would foretell the death of a member of the family. So if a single primrose was accidentally brought into the house then a member of the family would have to dance three times around the bloom to ward off any ill luck. Malicious neighbours would sometimes give a child a single primrose to take home, hoping this would result in bad fortune for that family. People carried this superstition even further. They would count the number of primroses growing in clumps in the garden, to make sure there were thirteen.

It was also thought unlucky to see a primrose flowering out of season, but it was considered lucky for a maid to pick a primrose surrounded by six leaves because this would help her find true love:

> The Primrose, when with six leaves gotten grace
> Maids, as a true love in their bosom place.

Primroses were also seen as a way of communication with the 'little people', like fairies and elves. In recognition of their powers and uncertain tempers, posies would be left on doorsteps to ask the fairies to bless the house and all those living there. Bunches of primroses would be hung up in cowsheds to encourage the fairies not to steal the milk. But if you wished to see the fairies, you had to eat the blooms.

Other uses including medicinal

The primrose has medicinal properties too. The leaves were pounded and made into a salve to use on wounds, and the dried and powdered roots were used to treat nervous disorders. It is still used by some people as an infusion to treat rheumatism, and as a general sedative or relaxant.

Annie Fry, an 84-year-old farmer's wife from Dorset, recalls how a long time ago a gypsy lady told her about a cure for skin complaints on the face. She was told to take three primrose leaves, boil them in one pint of water, and then drink the water. Unfortunately history does not relate whether or not this had the desired effect.

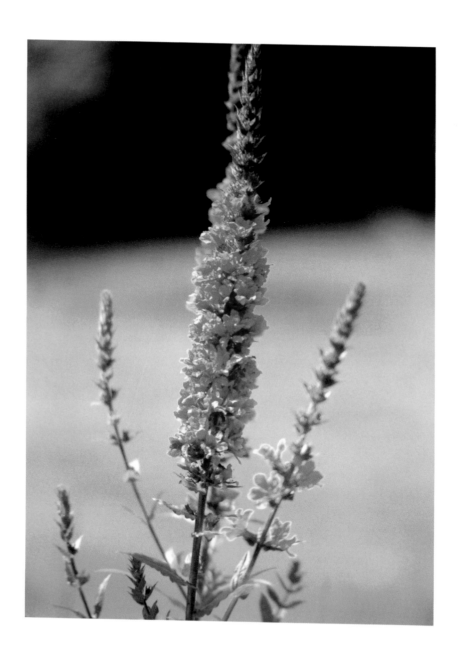

Purple Loosestrife

Purple Loosestrife
Llysiau'r Milwr Coch
Lythrum salicaria

Description
Purple loosestrife is a tall and colourful flower, with leaves growing in pairs or whorls round the stem. From June to August the bright reddish-purple six-petalled flowers can be seen in rings round the stem, just above the leaf whorls.

Habitat
This plant favours damp locations such as riverbanks, during the summer months of June to August. In damp fields in parts of Ireland, purple loosestrife and corn marigold can be seen flowering together. The combined colours create a beautiful sight.

Naming History
Originally grouped with the yellow loosestrife, *Lysmachia*, the generic name was mistranslated. The Roman naturalist Pliny stated that the plant was named after Lysimachos, the King of Thrace, Macedonia and Asia Minor, the supposed discoverer of the plant. But the Greek word *lysimachos* was wrongly translated as if from *luein*, (to loose) and *mache*, (stress), hence 'ending or calming stress' (loose strife) which also refers to some of its properties.

Other uses including medicinal
Because of its calming properties it was said to quieten irritable horses and oxen at the plough by being tied around their yokes. This was almost certainly because it warded off the biting flies and gnats, thereby offering them relief. This prompted John Gerard's quotation, "it appeases the strife and unrulinesse which falleth out among oxen at the plough, if it is put about their yokes, and the smoke of the burned herb drives away serpents and kills flies and gnats in the house".

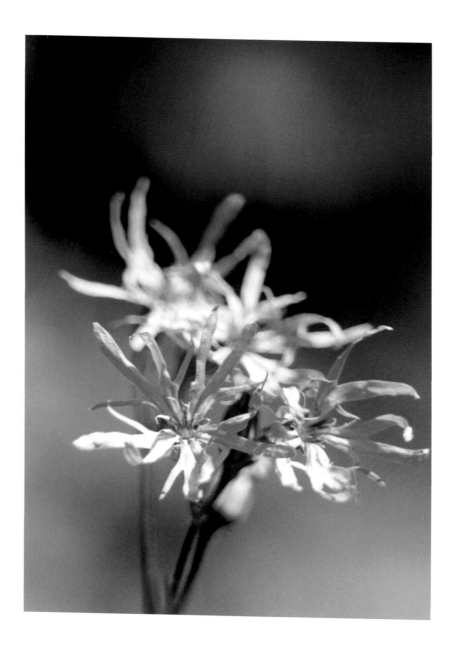

Ragged Robin

Ragged Robin
Blodau'r Brain, Ffrils y Merched
Lychnis flos-cuculi

Description

This is a curious and unmistakeable flower. Rough, slender stems of medium height support pairs of lanceolate leaves at intervals, and the pink flowers appear from May to August. The petals of these are each divided into four lobes, the splits reaching almost to the base of the petal and producing the characteristic 'ragged' appearance.

Habitat

Ragged Robin favours damp and marshy places, and is usually found growing among tall grasses or other plants that can help support the slender stem.

Naming History

Its common name is due to the plant's appearance, with its deep pink flowers each with deeply divided ragged petals. The generic name *Lychnis* originated from the Greek *lychnos*, 'lamp' and was probably so called because of the bright colour of the flowers. The specific name *flos-cuculi* means 'flower of the cuckoo', due to the fact that ragged robin flowers around the time that the cuckoo arrives. Other flowers share this privilege too along with cuckoo flower (lady's smock) *Cardamine pratensis*.

Folklore

In some country places during the time of Pentecost, travelling players would enact a farce called 'Robin and Marion'. Suggestions have been made that there could have been a link with the play and this plant and in the New Forest, the players were actually nick-named Ragged Robins.

Around the time of the sixteenth century, the buds of ragged robins were used for divination. Girls used to pick them and then give each one the name of a boy she liked, before placing them in her apron. The first one to open would bear the name of her future sweetheart. The poet Tennyson also used the name of Ragged Robin to describe a pretty damsel in ragged clothes.

Other uses including medicinal

Gerard had little to say about the plant's medical uses. "These are not used either in medicine or in nourishment," he wrote, "but they serve for garlands and crowns, and to decke up gardens". Despite this, ragged robin still brightens our countryside with its charm, lending colour and cheer where it grows.

Ragwort
Llysiau'r Gingroen
Senecio jacobaea

Description

Ragwort is a strong, self-supporting, medium to tall biennial plant. The leaves are deeply lobed, and the bright yellow, daisy-like flowers are composed of a number of florets. The flowers appear from June to October, and occur in dense clusters at the top of the plant.

Habitat

Common ragwort is at home in dry grassy places, waste ground, pastures and on roadsides throughout the British Isles.

Naming History

The name ragwort is often said to derive from the ragged shape of the plant's leaves, but it seems that this is completely wrong. In the sixteenth century a German *Herbal* was translated into English by somebody whose command of German was less than perfect. The German name *Ragwurz*, which was applied to this plant in an anglicised form, actually belonged to a species of orchid, and the mistake was perpetuated. The root 'rag' actually comes from a word meaning rampant sexual desire, as attributed to orchids since time immemorial. As far as is known, ragwort has no erotic or aphrodisiac qualities, and experimentation is not advisable, since it is in fact poisonous.

However, the ragwort's alternative name, 'St James's wort', is much more appealing. The connection with the saint is reflected in the specific name *jacobaea* and it is almost certainly attributed to St James, because it is in flower on St James's Day, 25th July.

The common and vernacular names associated with this plant are an indication of its status as an undesirable weed. One of the worst examples is the Scottish 'wee-bo', which translates as 'the little devil'. The vernacular name 'stinking Willie' comes from the nasty smelling leaves. In this case the 'Willie' referred to is the Duke of Cumberland, commonly known as the 'butcher', the victor of the battle of Culloden Moor. The legend says that the Ragwort was spread around by his Culloden campaign.

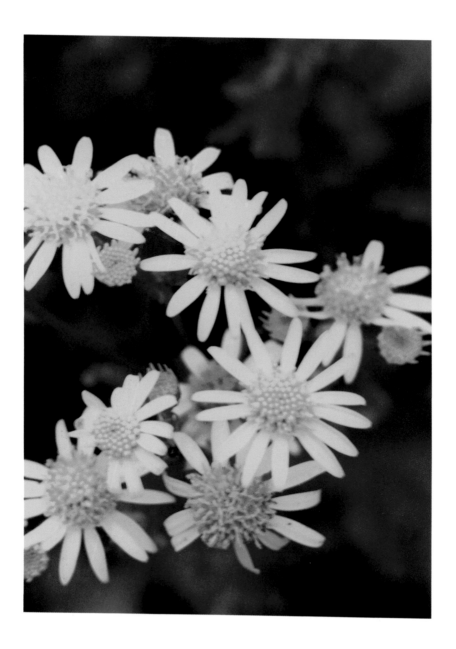

Ragwort

Folklore

Human nature being what it is, in some parts of the Highlands of Scotland a farmer who finished his harvesting first would take the last sheaf of corn cut from his field and make a small effigy of an old woman *(cailleach)*. He would dress this in docks and ragwort and give it to one of his neighbours who, more dilatory than him, had not yet finished the harvest. The doll represented an invisible hag whose powers would sap the resources of the slower reaper and jeopardise his chances over the coming winter. This, not unnaturally, was regarded as the act of an enemy among the crofters, and on occasion would give rise to bloodshed.

It is sometimes difficult to remember that a mediaeval villager would rarely, if ever, travel more than a few miles from his home. Consequently, the ability to fly freely from one place to another was often attributed to supernatural beings. Witches would fly on broomsticks, common objects about the house and fairies, being of lesser stature and inhabitants of the great outdoors, were reputed to ride the long, hard stalks of ragwort. By the sixteenth century, belief in fairies was dwindling fast and witches too were said to ride on ragwort stems. As Burns puts it:

> Let warlocks grim an' withered Hags
> Tell how wi' you on ragweed nags
> They skim the muirs on dizzy crags
> Wi 'wicked speed
> And in kirk-yards renew their leagues
> Owre howkit dead.

Other uses including medicinal

In several European countries ragwort is called 'St James's herb' and, because of its astringent juice, was once used to cure the sores and ulcers which afflicted the pilgrims who visited St James's shrine. The green leaves could be used in a poultice for the treatment of rheumatism, gout and sciatica while the root was pulverised and made into a decoction and used to treat internal bruising and general wounds. There are some references to the use of ragwort as a medicine for horses, as St James was the patron saint of horses. Another older name for ragwort is 'staggerwort', 'wort' meaning medicine and 'staggers' is an illness which affects horses. Never attempt this remedy. Ragwort is actually extremely poisonous to horses and can destroy their livers, although its foliage is bitter and animals will only eat it if they are very hungry. Even more dangerous is dried Ragwort if it gets in with the hay, because then it is more palatable but just as poisonous. It is wise to pull up all the ragwort in a field, before putting horses or cows in to pasture.

For centuries the plant has been used to make green, yellow and bronze dyes.

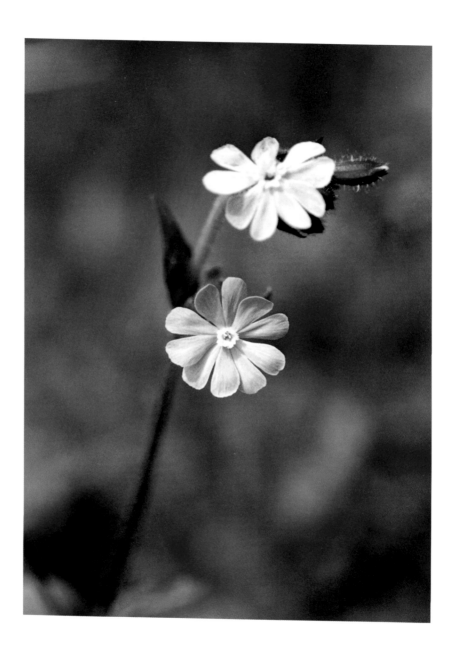

Red Campion

Red Campion
Llysiau'r Ychen, Ceiliog Coch
Silene dioica

Description

Red campion is a perennial of medium height, with a hairy stem and oval pointed leaves. The flowers, growing on stalks at the upper end of the plant, are variable in colour from dark pink through to pale pink. The five petals are slightly cleft at the ends. Red campion flowers from March to November.

Habitat

A very common flower, red campion can be found in fields, woods and shady hedges, particularly where generations of leaf mould have made the soil rich and nutritious.

Naming History

The word campion is from French and Latin origins meaning 'field', in terms of games and sports, and the modern word 'champion' is derived from it. This being so, it is not surprising to learn that these flowers (there is a white species as well) were once used to make chaplets or wreaths for crowning the winners of public games held on village greens in earlier times. A minor hazard of picking these flowers, which our ancestors will have experienced while making chaplets (and possibly while wearing them), is a sticky sap-like secretion often found on the stems. This may have the purpose of deterring voracious insects from climbing the stems to eat the leaves, and appears to be the origin of the generic name *Silene*, from the Greek *sialon*, 'saliva'.

Folklore

Buttons have long been a necessary part of clothing, but unfortunately require to be sown on to the garment, a complex procedure frequently considered (often with some justification) as being beyond the capabilities of men, particularly unmarried ones. Therefore some buttons were constructed in such a way as to resemble press studs and thus obviate the need for sewing. These unskilled, user-friendly devices were thus called 'bachelor's buttons'. In the seventeenth century especially, men's buttons were often surfaced with cloth, in bright colours and irregular shapes, and consequently various flowers were named bachelor's buttons by association. These included particularly red and white campions, white crowfoot and yellow buttercup.

In the words of Tennyson:

> In the spring a livelier iris changes on the burnish'd dove
> in the spring a young man's fancy lightly turns to thoughts of love.

Fortunately a less-than-confident young man would have the help of bachelor's buttons. He would keep a few of the red campion buds in his pocket, and if they opened it was an indication that he would find favour with his chosen girl. Wistful maidens would keep the buds beneath their aprons in the hope that they would be smiled upon by their fancied swains.

Other uses including medicinal

Other than its natural beauty, red campion does not appear to have any useful medicinal properties.

Red Clover
Meillion Coch
Trifolium pratense

Description

Usually low-growing, but sometimes quite tall when found in long grass, red clover has the familiar three-lobed leaves and globular pink flowerheads composed of a number of small florets. The flowers vary in colour from pink to purple and can be seen from May to October.

Habitat

The leaves of clover are a familiar sight in fields, road verges and lawns (much to the irritation of many gardeners).

Naming History

Red and white clover were broad distinguishing terms long before the Norman Conquest, but more or less generically the meadow clovers were taken to be grasses which happened to have flowers – flowers you could pick and pull off the petals and suck the ends for the sweet nectar.

The generic name *Trifolium* is a simple descriptive term meaning three-leaved. The origin of the common name is rather less clear. Apparently 'clover' comes from the earlier name 'claver' from the Latin word *clava* meaning 'club'. The allusion may not be immediately obvious until one thinks of a pack of cards, and the three-lobed clubs insignia. In fact the stylised clubs design was originally based on the club of Hercules, as seen in classical art, and bears a considerable resemblance to the clover leaf. Before 1600 the name 'claver' was more commonly used than the more modern name of 'clover'. This gave rise to some of the place names that we know today, such as Claverdon, or 'Clover Hill', in Warwickshire and Claverton, 'Clover Farmstead', in Cheshire.

Folklore

Clovers, especially four-leaved clovers, have for generations been associated with good luck. To say that someone is in clover, means that he is in luck or prosperous, like cows feeding in a field of clover. Clover is related to lucerne which is grown as cattle fodder, a food that cows relish. Clover was used in love divination, so not surprisingly to dream about it was thought to signify a happy marriage.

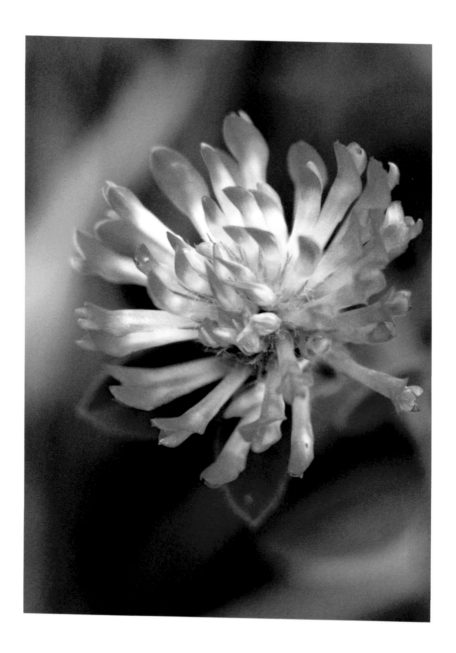

Red Clover

A clover, a clover or two
Put it in your right shoe
The first young man (or woman) you meet,
In field, lane or street,
You shall have him, (or her) or one of their name.

The four-leaved clover was thought to give the possessor the power to see fairies, as well as bringing them good luck. In fact a story about a Northumberland milkmaid returning from the pasture after milking, says that she saw a group of fairies dancing in the grass. On examination it was discovered that the grass pad that she was wearing on her head, as protection from the milkpail, contained a four-leaved clover.

Many wild flowers are associated with Christianity and the triple-leaved clover was linked with the Holy Trinity. Maybe it was used by monks and priests, to explain this doctrine to people in the past. A four-leaved clover was thought to detect witches and provide safety from all evil. Therefore a four-leaved clover hidden in the cowshed was thought to protect the cows from evil magic and ensure that the cows yielded good rich milk to make better quality butter.

Other uses including medicinal

Clover belongs to a group of plants known as nitrogen-fixers, which have the property of enriching the soil with nitrates, thus fertilizing it. In farming practice it has been common since the middle ages to grow a crop of clover or related plant every few years, thereby improving the soil and getting a better yield from the next crop grown there. The clover can be used as a cattle fodder.

Again the Welsh demonstrate their fondness for infusions as they used to collect and dry the leaves naturally out of direct sunlight and then make a tea with them which they believed reduced consumption.

The four-leaved clover shape is often employed today for motorway junctions. It provides an easy and convenient pattern for cars to leave one motorway and join another without crossing traffic streams.

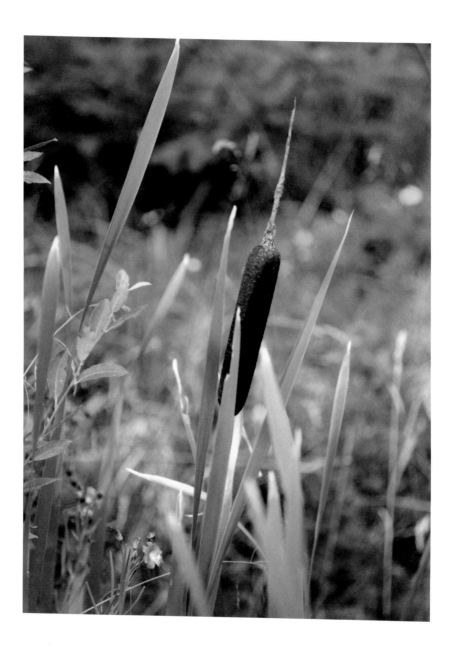

Reedmace

Reedmace
Typha latifolia

Description

Reedmace has long narrow greyish leaves and long chocolate-brown spear-shaped flowers about 10-15cm long. It can be seen flowering in damp conditions during the summer months of June and July. At the end of the flowering period, the brown seed pod bursts to release the soft fluffy thistledown-like seeds to the summer breezes.

Habitat

Reedmace favours water margins, particularly ponds and lakes where the water is shallow and silty, and is usually found growing in the shallows.

Naming History

The well known picture of Moses in the Bulrushes, could equally well be called 'Moses in the Reedmace'. The name 'bulrush' is indiscriminately applied to various species, particularly this one, and the completely dissimilar club-rushes (*Scirpus lacustris*), and confusion has arisen.

Folklore

A Welsh folk story tells about King March ap Meirchion who lived near Abersoch in Llyn. He suffered a great embarrassment; he had ears like a horse. No one knew about his secret except for his barber, whom he had sworn to silence. Eventually the king told his plight to a physician, who told him to whisper his secret to the earth. He went away and did as he had been told, and to his surprise beautiful tall reeds sprang up. One day some musicians passed by on their way to entertain at the court of King Maelgwn Gwynedd at Castell March. One of them saw the reeds and cut one of them to make himself a new pipe, which he played before the king, but it would only play 'March ap Meirchion has horse's ears'. Following that incident, the king never again complained about his very large ears.

In a later version of the tale, King March ap Meirchion is said to have killed each of his barbers, and buried their bodies under the earth where the fine reeds grew.

Another story tells of a severe fish famine in Conwy. One day St Bride was walking along the river throwing rushes into the water, and at the same time praying for an end to the famine. A few days later, the rushes were mysteriously transformed into fish. In no time the river teemed with fish again who have since been known as 'brwyniaid' (sparlings) meaning 'rushlike'.

Other uses including medicinal

The soft seeds or down used to be gathered by country people and used to stuff mattresses. It must have taken a very large quantity of down to stuff one mattress, and presumably only the most dedicated slug-a-bed would have taken the trouble to do so.

Unlike the down, the leaves are tough, pliable and waterproof, and have been used for many purposes where these qualities are necessary, especially in making baskets and small coracle-like boats. How leakproof these were is unrecorded, but they would at least have had the merit of being cheap for lakeside dwellers. These days the flowers are much used in floral decorations.

Nowadays when conservationists are managing wetlands, reedmace is one of the prime species to be planted in order to stabilise the marsh and increase the species diversity.

Ribwort Plantain
Plantago lanceolata

Description
Most people will be familiar with the plantain. The flat rosette of tough leaves can stand being trodden on or driven over without damage, but the brown, oval-shaped flowers with a dusting of whitish anthers grow on erect stalks, rather resembling a grass flower.

Habitat
Plantains grow in waste and stony ground, sports fields, car parks and otherwise well-tended lawns.

Naming History
The specific name *lanceolata* (spear-shaped) comes from the fact that the leaves of this plant are long and gradually tapering. They also have prominent parallel veins running the full length of the leaf, which accounts for the common name of 'ribwort'. The generic name *Plantago* is thought to have come down from the Latin *planta*, 'sole' (meaning of the foot), because the basal leaves resemble the shape of a footprint, and because of their tolerance to being trodden on.

The hard flowerhead on a tough stalk has for centuries been known by names such as 'soldier' or 'fighting cock', and games similar to conkers have been played by children for generations, matching one 'hardhead' against another until one loses its head. These games are common across Europe as well as Britain, and local names reflect this. In Somerset you may find 'swords and spears', and in Scotland 'soldier's tappie', among many others.

Folklore
Belligerence, however, is not the only characteristic of the plantain. Since time immemorial, farmers have been concerned about fire in their hayricks. Paradoxically, a wet rick is more likely to burn than a dry one, since the moisture in the centre will cause fermentation, giving rise to heat. In the centre of a rick, this heat will be trapped and will build up to the point where the rick will catch fire spontaneously. The leaves of the plantain were once known as 'fire-leaves' and an experienced farmer would twist the leaves in his hands to see how moist they were, using this as guidance to the amount of moisture in the hay and thus the likelihood of ignition.

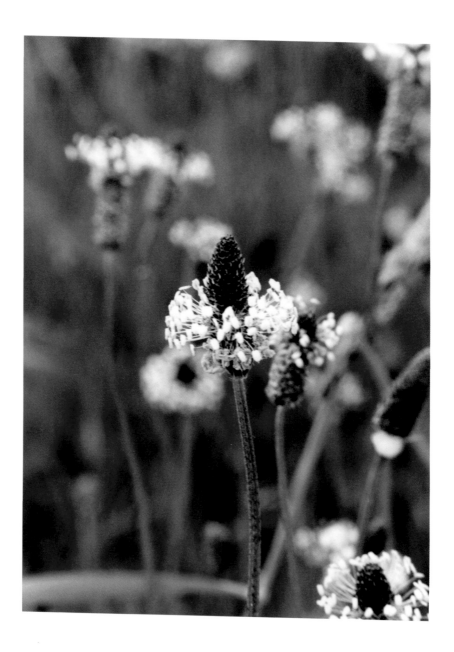

Ribwort Plantain

Other uses including medicinal

The Anglo-Saxons had their own uses for plantains. It was believed that if carried on the person it would 'withstand evil and vile things and all the loathsome ones that through the land rove', and, perhaps more practically, that if bound to the head with red wool, it would cure headaches. Counter-productively, it can also generate hay fever in those unlucky enough to be allergic to its pollen, and for them a different headache cure would be advisable.

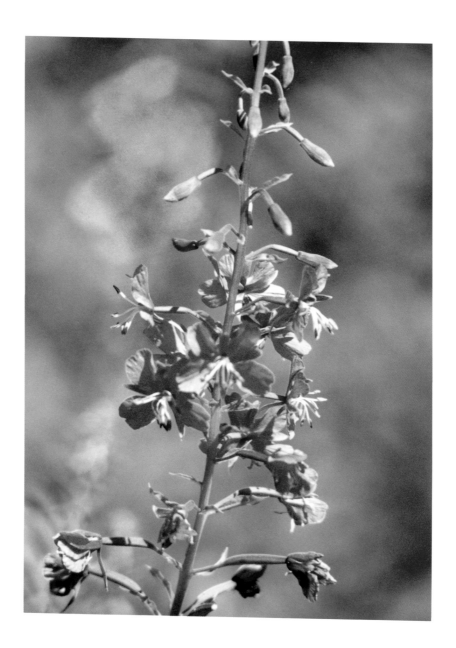

Rosebay Willowherb

Rosebay Willowherb
Llysiau Santes Fair
Epilobium angustifolium

Description

John Gerard, the English herbalist and barber-surgeon (1545-1612), was very fond of rosebay willowherb and grew it in his garden. He described it as being "very goodly to behold, for the decking up of houses and gardens. The branches come out of the ground in great numbers, growing to the height of sixe foote, garnished with brave flowers of great beautie, consisting of fower leaves a piece, of an orient purple colour. The cod is long... and full of downie matter, which flieth away with the winde when the cod is opened." This last sentence refers to the long, slender seedpod, which opens to reveal a mass of thistledown-like leaves.

Habitat

Rosebay willowherb is one of the largest and most spectacular of our wild flowers, and is a familiar sight in open woods, on heaths, on waste ground and even on mountainsides. It grows in large patches and, when in bloom, a broad expanse of the pink blossom resembles a large area of blazing fire. It is one of the first colonisers of bare and disturbed ground, and after the Blitz on London in the Second World War it grew prolifically on bomb sites

Naming History

The French for this plant is '*herbe de Saint-Antoine*', or 'St Anthony's fire', after its habit of colonising bomb sites and large areas of waste ground. The specific name *angustifolium* means 'narrow leaved' which – as the leaves are very similar to the willow – explains the common name of this family of plants: the willowherbs.

Other uses including medicinal

Nicholas Culpeper also liked this plant for its medical properties. He described it as being a plant of Saturn, cooling and astringent. The fresh juice or the powdered root can be taken to stop internal haemorrhaging. It stops "looseness of the bowel and other fluxes and also nocturnal pollutions". In modern uses the herb, dried and infused, is used in the treatment of whooping cough and asthma. In Europe, rosebay willowherb leaves were dried and used as an astringent tea, and in Siberia, an alcoholic drink has been made using this herb and the fly agaric mushroom!

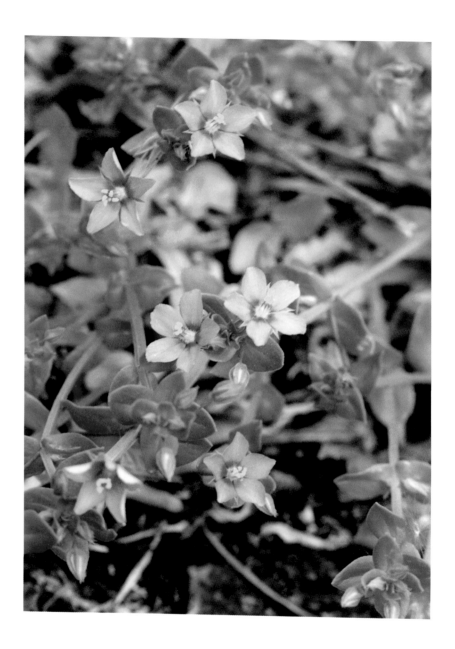

Scarlet Pimpernel

Scarlet Pimpernel
Llysiau'r Cryman, Coch yr ŷd, Gwlydd Mair
Anagallis arvensis

Description

This little annual plant is usually described as 'prostrate' meaning that it is a creeping plant which grows close to the ground. The stems are square and the leaves are oval, and the flowers, which are usually red, may be paler orange or even pink. They grow from the leaf bases and open in sunlight, and may be seen from May to October.

Habitat

Almost any time during the summer, you may take a walk along a lane or a hedge, particularly where the ground is fairly dry, and find the small orange-red stars of scarlet pimpernel. It is sometimes called a weed of cultivation, and may be found where the soil is disturbed and then left.

Naming History

The roots of the name pimpernel are very confusing. It appears to mean 'pepper-like' and burnet saxifrage was once called pimpernel since the fruits resembled small peppers. So far, so good. As it happens burnet saxifrage leaves are rather similar to scarlet pimpernel leaves and non botanically minded people transferred the name to scarlet pimpernel, not realising it was a different plant, and the name stuck. The word has other possible sources, however. An old French word *pimper* meant 'smart', or 'trim', and this could be held to apply to this flower. Alternatively the Welsh word 'pump' (pronounced 'pimp') means five and these small attractive flowers have five petals. Whether the Welsh name would have influenced the English one is open to question.

> Al day ageyn undern and non
> He wyl bym spredyn and on-don,
> And ageyne the ewene-tyde
> He lokyth hym-self be every syde;
> He growyth be the erthe lowe,
> Nyh every man wyl hym knowe.

These lines from a mediaeval poem date from about 1400. Due to their sensitivity to temperature and humidity the flowers open in the sun and close when it is about to rain, giving rise to the name of 'shepherd's weatherglass' or 'poor man's weatherglass'.

As well as being sensitive to moisture, the flowers open every day at about eight in the morning and close about mid-afternoon, and could be used as a rudimentary rustic clock.

The generic name for scarlet pimpernel *Anagallis* is possibly descended from the Greek *anagelao* meaning 'I laugh', due to the fact that it was once believed that these plants could be beneficial in the treatment of depression, thus giving it the names of 'laughter bringer', 'shepherd's joy' and 'shepherd's delight'. Some other attractive country names include 'change in the weather' from Norfolk, 'grandfather's weatherglass' from Cornwall and 'John-go-to-bed-at-noon' from Somerset. A Welsh name that generates from the sixteenth century was 'gwlydd Mair', 'Mary's stalk'.

Folklore

In 1905 Baroness Orczy wrote the well-known novel *The Scarlet Pimpernel*. This was the romantic story of an English nobleman, Sir Percy Blakeney, who, under the codename of 'Scarlet Pimpernel', rescued many French aristocrats from the guillotines of the French Revolution. He apparently called himself after one of the smaller and least conspicuous flowers that would be known to the Baroness' audience.

For some reason, it was once said that if you dropped a scarlet pimpernel into running water, it would move against the current, but why this should be is not recorded. On a rather more practical note, holding a flower in your hand was believed to give you second sight and hearing and would enable you to understand the speech of birds and animals.

Other uses including medicinal

Scarlet pimpernel was a useful herb against a variety of conditions, such as toothache and snake bite, inflammation of the kidney, liver problems and also as an antidepressant. In the eighteenth century it was considered useful in the treatment of hydrophobia.

The leaves of the scarlet pimpernel can give some people dermatitis.

Selfheal
Craith Unnos
Prunella vulgaris

Description
Selfheal is a member of the labiate family, which includes peas and beans, hence the characteristic shape of the two-lobed, purple flowers. It is a low-creeping perennial with pointed oval leaves, the flowers growing in spikes or clusters from June to November.

Habitat
Selfheal grows in grassy places and on bare ground, and not infrequently in uncut lawns!

Naming History
The common name indicates that this plant had many medicinal uses and was considered useful as a wound herb. Its generic name *Prunella* is from the German word *brunella*, the old name for 'quinsy', a severe form of tonsillitis, for which this plant was used to heal the symptoms. In fact Cole, a seventeenth-century, writer said that the throat-shaped flowers of Selfheal indicated that it was beneficial for the relief of throat problems. Another suggestion states that the name could have come from another German word *braun* meaning brown, because of the dark brown colour of the seeding heads.

Other uses including medicinal
The common name selfheal implies that anyone who is ill may be able to cure themselves by using the properties of this plant. So much so in fact that both John Gerard (1545-1612) – the English herbalist whose London garden became famous for its rare plants – and Nicholas Culpeper recommended it as a wound herb on account of its astringent properties. Culpeper describes it in his herbal as taken in syrups for inward wounds and used in unguents and on plasters for outward wounds. He wrote that it was good for washing wounds with and for injecting into ulcers, and where sores, ulcers, inflammations or swellings needed to be repressed, it was also effective. It helped to "cleanse the foulness of sores and speedily heal them". It was a very effective remedy for fresh wounds, he said, because it "stays the flux of blood from the wound and solders up the lips. It will

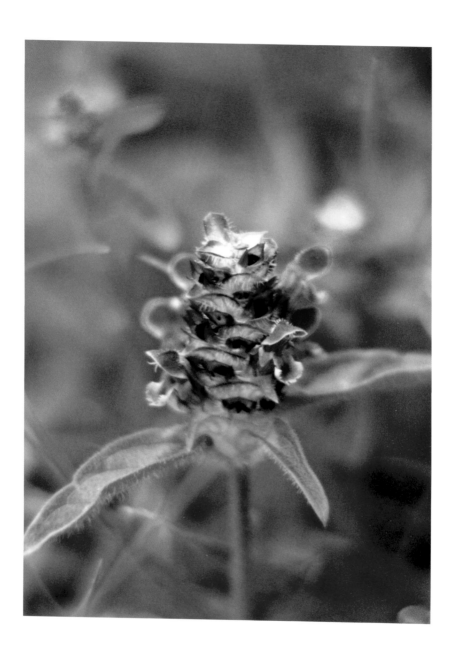

Selfheal

remove a headache, if the temples and forehead are anointed with the juice mixed with the Oil of Roses. Also the same mixed with honey from roses, cleanses and heals ulcers in the mouth and throat as well as those in the 'secret parts'."

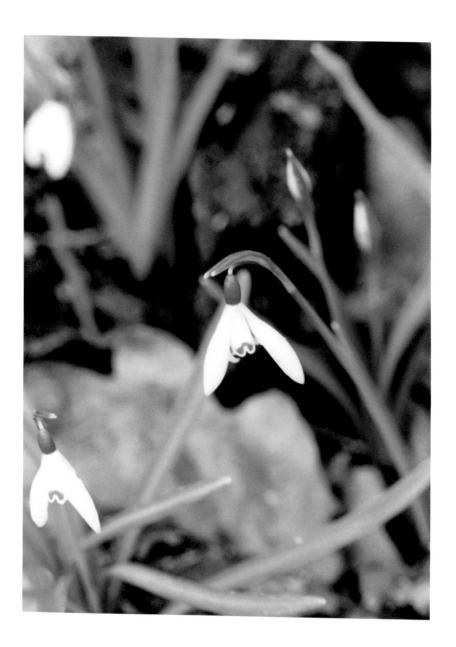

Snowdrop

Snowdrop
Eirlys, Cloch Maban
Galanthus nivalis

Description

A very familiar short perennial plant, the snowdrop has a clump of bright green fleshy leaves growing from the base, and white, nodding, bell-shaped flowers on individual stems. These arise between January and March, before the other plants of the woodland floor start to emerge.

Habitat

The snowdrop is always the first to appear after the long winter months, an attractive and welcome sight clustered around the base of a tree, or growing in carpets in damp woods, beside shady streams, meadows and extensively along the roadsides of north Wales in early spring. In fact wild snowdrops were first recorded in the 1770s, growing in the counties of Gloucestershire and Worcestershire.

Naming History

The common name refers to the colour and drop-like shape of the flowers, similar to the 'drop-like' pearl pendants worn by the ladies of the sixteenth and seventeenth centuries. The generic name *Galanthus* comes from the Greek *gala* meaning 'milk' and *anthos* meaning 'flower', whereas the specific name *nivalis* simply means 'snow-white', or 'growing near snow'.

Although they may or may not be native, snowdrops grew in Elizabethan gardens and used to be called bulbous violets. In fact Sir Thomas Hanmer mentions them in his *Garden Book* which he wrote in 1659. "Bulbous violets... whose pretty pure white bellflowers are tipped a fine greene, and hang downe their heads." It wasn't until the end of the seventeenth century that snowdrop was used as the common name. But it looks as if the name snowdrop had originally come from the German *Schneetropfen* or Swedish *snodroppe*, the latter by obvious association of ideas.

Folklore

The Victorians regarded snowdrops as a symbol of hope, as they were one of the first flowers to appear each year. They also believed that because these flowers grew so close to the bare earth, they were therefore associated with death, and close to those who were dead and buried. It was therefore considered bad luck to bring a single bloom into the house, because this could cause the death of a member of the family before the year was out. In some areas, however, a whole bunch of blooms was considered to be quite safe. Legends also say that happiness comes to a house where snowdrops grow beneath the windows, and a planted bowl of snowdrops placed in a room was said to do no harm.

The traditional feast of Candlemas has long been held on 2nd February. In the church calendar it was once known as the Feast of the Purification of the Virgin Mary and snowdrops, often being in flower at that time and white in colour, were associated with this festival and known as Candlemas bells. The association of the colour white with virginity also meant that young girls wore them as protection from overly amorous young men.

An attractive legend states that the snowdrop became a symbol of hope when Adam and Eve were expelled from the Garden of Eden. Apparently Eve was about to give up hope that the cold winters would ever end, when an angel appeared, and transformed some of the snowflakes into snowdrops, proving that the winters do eventually end and give way to spring.

Soft Rush
Brwynen, Pabwyren
Juncus effusus

Description
Soft rush can be easily recognised by its smooth glossy stems, lack of proper leaves and compact brownish flower heads. Unlike ordinary flowers, the outer green layer of the stems can be peeled to reveal the spongy white pith within.

Habitat
Soft rush is commonly found growing in wet marshy areas or near water.

Folklore
In some churches a Sunday (generally near the festival of the saint to whom the church was dedicated) was laid aside to renew the rushes which covered the church floor. This custom is still carried out at St Mary Redcliffe in Bristol, on Whit Sunday and at Ambleside in Grasmere and elsewhere in Westmorland. At Ambleside, a rush-bearing procession is held on the Saturday nearest St Anne's Day (26th July), the church being dedicated to St Anne. This festival is known as Rush-bearing Sunday.

In the days when floors used to be strewn with rushes, important guests were given clean rushes, whereas those of inferior standing were left with used rushes or none at all, hence the phrase 'not worth a rush'.

Other uses including medicinal
True candles made with wax were far too expensive for many people to afford and the 'rush dip' was a barely acceptable but much cheaper substitute.

To ensure a supply of lights through the winter, rushes would be cut in summer and stored in water. When needed they would be peeled, leaving one thin strip to hold the pith together, and then dipped in grease. This grease was obtained from the dripping fat while meat was cooked, and collected in a long shallow vessel, known as a 'gresset', or 'cresset'. Here it would be stored until needed for candle-making. The gresset would be warmed enough to liquefy the grease and a strip of pith would be dipped in this repeatedly, to build up solid layers, the pith acting as the wick. When the rush dip thus produced was suffi-ciently thick, it would be held horizontally in a metal clamp and one or both ends would be lit. The light it gave would be dim, yellow and smoky, and no doubt it would have dripped hot fat generously, but it would have enabled work to go on in the house after dark. The phrase 'burning the candle at both ends', signifying activity late at night, whether work or play, comes from the practice of lighting both ends of a rush dip to gain extra light. Gilbert White in the *Natural History of Selborne* estimated that a pound and a half of rushes would last a family for a year, at a cost of 4s 6d.

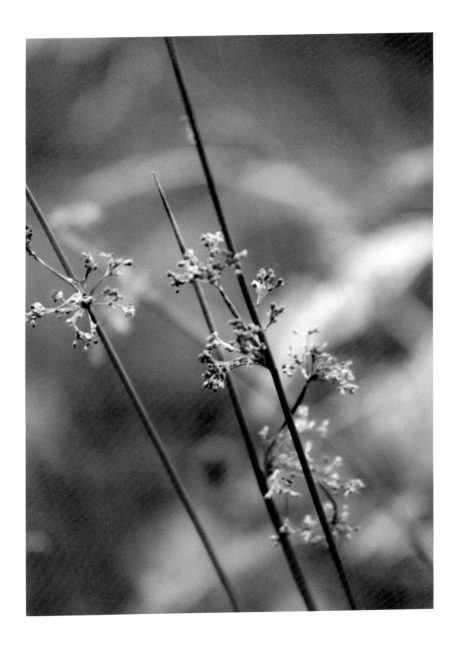

Soft Rush

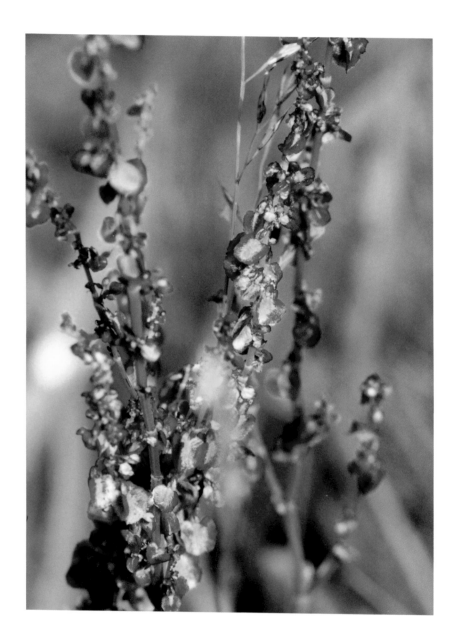

Sorrel

Sorrel
Dail Surion Bach
Rumex acetosa

Description

At first sight, common sorrel may not be recognised as a flower at all. The tall thin spike with tiny reddish-brown flowers clustered up it resembles a grass head, and it is only on closer inspection that the blooms can be seen to be true flowers. This confusion is compounded because common sorrel can often be found in grassy areas. The leaves, however, are quite conventional, being long and fairly narrow with slightly wavy edges and a pronounced midrib. The flowers occur from May to August and are followed by the seeds which at a casual glance appear very similar.

Habitat

Common sorrel is a familiar sight growing in the long grass of meadows, woods and roadside verges. It is not affected by the type of soil it grows in.

Naming History

When William Turner wrote his famous herbal in 1538 he gave the names *sorell* and *sourdoc* to this plant. Sorell came from the old French *surele,* in turn from *sur* which also means sour. Both these names refer to the sharp taste of the leaves.

Other uses including medicinal

Common sorrel was mainly used as a culinary plant. It has a cooling acid taste, similar to lemons, and was used to make a pleasant green sauce to go with fish. This sauce was made by pulping the leaves and mixing them with sugar and vinegar. In addition to this the leaves could be boiled in a little water and be served with pork, or with goose as an alternative to apple sauce. John Gerard (1545-1612) was an English herbalist and barber-surgeon born in Nantwich. He was author of *The Herball or General Historie of Plantes*, and his London garden was well renowned for its rare plants. He was particularly complimentary about the virtues of sorrel leaves and said that "The juice hereof in summer time is a profitable sauce in many meates, and pleasant to the taste. It cooleth an hot stomacke; moveth appetite to meate; tempereth the heate of the liver, and openeth the stoppings thereof."

The juice from the leaves could also be used for taking the rust marks out of linen, and an attractive reddish-brown dye could be obtained from the flowers, which was useful for colouring clothes. A horse of a bright chestnut colour is sometimes called a sorrel.

Despite being used for culinary purposes, sorrel does in fact contain a small quantity of poisonous oxalic acid. Also known as salts of sorrel, this was used as a household cleanser and if swallowed accidentally, one recommended antidote was tablespoon doses of plaster taken from the walls, powdered and mixed with water. The plaster would have been alkaline, and would have served to neutralise the acid. In passing to reassure anyone who may be fond of sorrel leaves, you would need to consume about a hundred-weight before noticing the effects of the poison.

Stinging Nettle
Danadl Poethion
Urtica dioica

Description

One of the first plants that many people learn to recognise as children, the stinging nettle is, fortunately, fairly distinctive. Variable in height (it may grow to more than a metre) the stiff, fibrous stem supports pointed oval leaves at frequent intervals. The leaves are serrated on the edges. The stings resemble short, fine hairs in appearance and occur on the stems as well as the leaves. The flowers are rather catkin-like in appearance, grow in feathery sprays from the bases of the leaves and are a pale cream to green in colour. It is said that nettles do not sting when they are in flower, but in fact this refers to the similar but unarmed dead nettle, so don't take the chance. Nettles spread through their roots, so tend to grow in large clumps.

Habitat

Nettles like growing on nitrogen-rich soils and are related to hemp, and surprisingly enough fig and mulberry. They are one of the commonest weeds and will grow anywhere, on waste ground or where the ground is left untenanted, even in gardens. It is a valuable food plant for several of our more colourful butterflies, especially the small tortoiseshell (*Aglais urtica*) whose caterpillars feed exclusively on nettles.

Naming History

Everyone recognises stinging nettles and nearly everyone must have been stung by one at sometime in their life. Although the origin of the name 'nettle' is rather more obscure, it may derive from the Anglo-Saxon word 'noedl', meaning needle because of the sharp needle-like shape of the stings. The sting itself is a modified hair and resembles a minute hypodermic needle, made of silica. It is hollow and contains a small amount of poison. When touched the tip breaks, and the sharp edges of the needle penetrate the skin and the poison is injected into the unwary. The pain is familiar to all and the subsequent itching rash is called *urticaria* from the generic name *Urtica* which comes from the Latin *urere*, to burn.

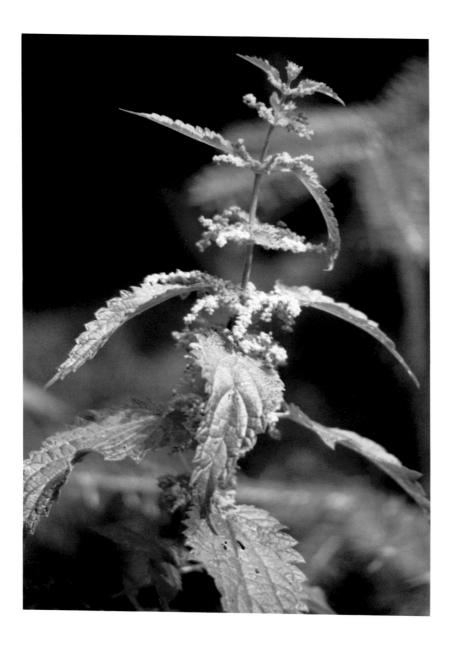

Stinging Nettle

Folklore

Unaware that the nettle flourishes in the temperate north European climate, Roman soldiers carried nettle seeds to sow. Due to the damp weather and their doubtless rather unsuitable clothing, the Romans suffered a lot from rheumatism, so they whipped their rheumaticky joints to stimulate the blood flow and relieve the pain. Consequently they took their own nettles with them on campaign, which resulted in the widespread growth of several different races of nettle.

In past times country people were very afraid of lightning, as this could set fire to their crops, or to the thatched roofs of their houses. They went to considerable lengths to protect themselves from the elements, and this included strewing nettles around the house, or throwing them on the fire, as they thought this would ward off lightning during a storm.

Other uses including medicinal

At the beginning of the First World War, thousands of men joined the army and this rose to millions over the next five years. These men had to be provided with uniforms. Nettle stalks supplied a coarse thread and, in order to save on cotton, this could be used to make army shirts. With careful dressing this could be made almost as fine as silk, although it is unlikely this applied to military requirements. Indeed legend had it that the manufacturers did not even bother to remove the stings...

Nettles also had many domestic uses; oil can be extracted from nettles and this too was useful. Nettle oil was used in lamps before paraffin was invented and, because of its availability, nettle juice was also used to curdle milk instead of rennet in cheesemaking. Also nettle juice combed through the hair was thought to be a cure for baldness. Fruit which had been packed in nettles was found to retain its bloom and the juice was used to seal cracks in wooden tubs and barrels. Nettles were also used to increase laying in hens. (Whether they were placed underneath the hen I do not know, but I am sure that would make them lay all right.) Bunches of nettles used to be hung up in the larders to keep away flies, and hung near beehives to deter frogs!

In medical terms however, Culpeper believed that nettle seeds offered an antidote against the stinging of venomous creatures, the biting of mad dogs, the poisonous qualities of hemlock, henbane, nightshade, mandrake or similar herbs that dull the senses.

For many years nettle juice has been drunk as a tonic, and there is an old rhyme which advises:

> Sup Nettles in March and Mugwort in May
> And many fair ladies won't go to the clay.

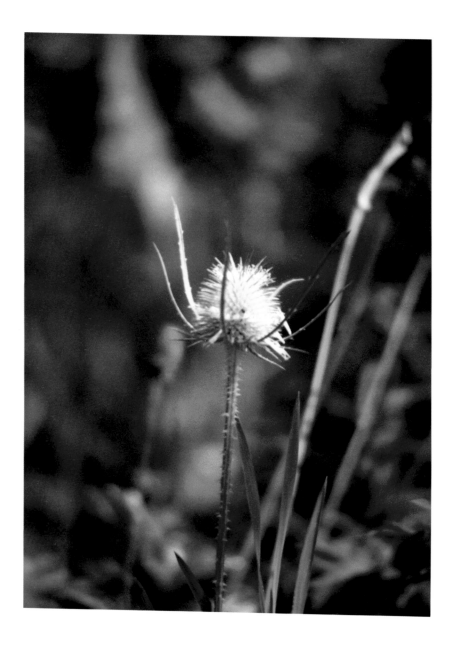

Teasel

Teasel
Llysiau'r Cribau, Llysiau'r Creigiau
Dipsacus fullonum

Description
This tall stately plant flowers during the summer months of July and August. The flowers are pale purple and cover the ovoid spiny head. These flowers then become dry fruiting heads in the autumn and are a favourite food of seed-eating birds like goldfinches. The stems are stiff and spiny, as are the leaves, and are usually cupped at the base, forming a basin around the stem in which water collects.

Habitat
Teasel grows in bare and grassy places, sometimes in damp conditions. The dead stems and flowerheads are persistent, and can be seen all winter when other vegetation has died back.

Naming History
The common name teasel comes from the Anglo-Saxon word *taesan* meaning 'to tease', because the dry seed heads were used for brushing over or 'teasing' the wool or cloth to raise the nap (the fibres).

Another country name for Teasel was 'shepherd's rod'. Possibly the tall stiff spiny stem resembled a shepherd's crook, or maybe a shepherd might find the stalk useful for prodding sheep at suitable times and suitable places. The Romans called the teasel *labrum Veneris*, 'lip of Venus', or *lavacrum Veneris*, 'basin of Venus' because of the way the leaves join around the stem and hold rain water. How this should benefit the plant is unclear.

Other uses including medicinal
In woollen mills, it was necessary to treat the newly woven cloth. To produce a smooth or rough surface as required, teasels would be placed into the wooden frames for combing the cloth to raise the nap or fibres. This process was carried out by workers known as 'fullers', hence the specific name of *fullonum*. A particular variety known as fuller's teasel was used for this purpose, because the bracts curve backwards, making them easier to use for this application.

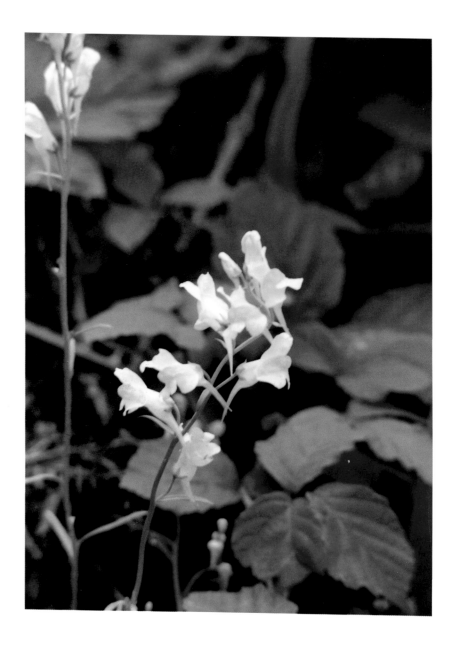

Toadflax

Toadflax
Llin y Llyffant, Trwyn y Llo
Linaria vulgaris

Description
The leaves of this common toadflax are linear in shape and untoothed, and grow numerously up the stem, giving the plant the resemblance of flax. The flowers, which appear throughout the summer from June to October, are yellow with an orange spot on the lower lip, and have a long straight spur. They grow in stalked spikes at the head of the stem.

Habitat
Common toadflax can be found growing in small patches on bare ground and waste places.

Naming History
Toadflax is sometimes called 'snapdragons', because when children gently squeeze the side of the flowers, the lower lip opens and shuts like a dragon's mouth. It is uncertain why the prefix 'toad' was applied, although it seems that this plant was originally used to treat festering swellings or 'buboes', and this may have become confused with the Latin for toad, *bufo*. Reinforcing this argument is the fact that the skin of a toad is covered with warty swellings resembling 'bubos' and the name of the plant may have been adopted from either direction. Also the leaves do look rather like flax and toadflax was a weed found in flax and could easily be mistaken for it until the flowers appeared. So it was named *Linaria* (*linum* meaning 'flax') and the Germans gave it the name of '*Krotenflacks*', which was translated later into 'todesflax' by William Turner in 1548. The apothecaries had their own name for toadflax, '*urinalis*', on account of this plant having some reputation of being a diuretic as well as the colour of the flowers.

Never allow toadflax to grow in your garden, it is a very tenacious weed and only needs a quarter of an inch of root to grow a new plant. It was introduced into the USA, where it was given the names of 'brideweed', 'butter and eggs', 'impudent lawyer' and, very appropriately, 'rabbit-flower'. The Norwegians call it 'torskemund', 'cod's mouth', maybe for the same reason as the name 'snapdragons', whereas the English names of 'eggs and bacon' and 'butter and eggs', obviously refer to the orange and yellow colours of the flowers.

Other uses including medicinal

As mentioned above, the apothecaries used to call toadflax '*urinalis*', because of the yellow colour of the flowers, and the fact that this plant could be used as a diuretic.

Vetch
Pys Llygod
Vicia cracca

Description
Vetch is a slender, clambering plant, with a stem that is unable to support its own weight. It compensates for this by using tendrils, which twine round the stems of adjacent plants, to climb up to the sunlight. The leaves are pinnate, meaning that they consist of pairs of leaflets on a common stalk, which ends in a tendril. The flowers are small, purple and lipped. Vetch flowers from June to August.

Habitat
Vetch prefers a dry habitat, usually bare or grassy ground or hedgerows.

Naming History
Vetches are climbing, binding plants, and most species possess tendrils which they use to climb up other plants. This is illustrated by both the common name 'vetch' and the generic name *Vicia* which are thought to have come from the Latin *vincio*, meaning 'I bind'.

There are many different species of vetch, and I mention just a few:

Horseshoe vetch, *Hippocrepis comosa,* is so called because the pods are arranged in a horseshoe shape, which is illustrated by both the common and generic names. *Hippocrepis* comes from the Greek *hippos* 'horse' and *crepis*, 'shoe'. The specific name *comosa* means 'tufted'.

Bush vetch (pys y berth, *Vicia sepium)* is so called because the common name describes a climbing, entwining plant, where the flowers form dense bushy clumps. The specific name *sepium* simply means 'of hedgerows'.

Kidney vetch (pys yr aren, *Anthyllis vulneraria),* is so-called because, as the common name suggests, it is a plant with vetch-like flowers, but has kidney-shaped lower leaves. It also had an early medicinal use in treating kidney disorders, and was used as a wound herb. This is indicated by the specific name *vulneraria* meaning 'wound healing'. The generic name *Anthyllis* is believed to have come from *anthos,* a Greek word meaning 'flower' and *ioulos*, 'down', because the flowers are slightly downy.

Bitter vetch (pys y maes, *lathyrus montanus L.*) is the only vetch eaten by humans. In the sixteenth century in northern Scotland and the Hebrides, the tuberous rhizomes were dug up and eaten. On the Isle of Colonsay they ate them fresh and raw, without even bothering to cook them. They also tied them up in bundles, and dried them under the thatch. They even used them for flavouring whisky. Gerard, who enjoyed eating the rhizomes, likened the taste to chestnuts.

Folklore

The vetch family was originally introduced by farmers for cattle fodder, and is thought to have come from western Asia. In the early eighteenth century, Miller wrote in his *Gardener's Dictionary*, that 'common vetch' *Vicia sativa* was cultivated in the fields for the seed, which is the common food of pigeons. Grown for early fodder, vetches have now naturalised themselves throughout the British Isles.

In Europe the vetch is called the 'tare', and this has led many people to believe that it was the tare of the Bible, growing as a weed in the cornfields and destined to be hurled into the furnace at harvest time, while the good grain was stored. This has been disputed and another school of thought declares that 'tare' was, in fact, the darnel grass. You pays your money and takes your choice... They are very hardy plants, and an old saying from the mid eighteenth century says:

A vetch will grow through
The bottom of an old shoe.

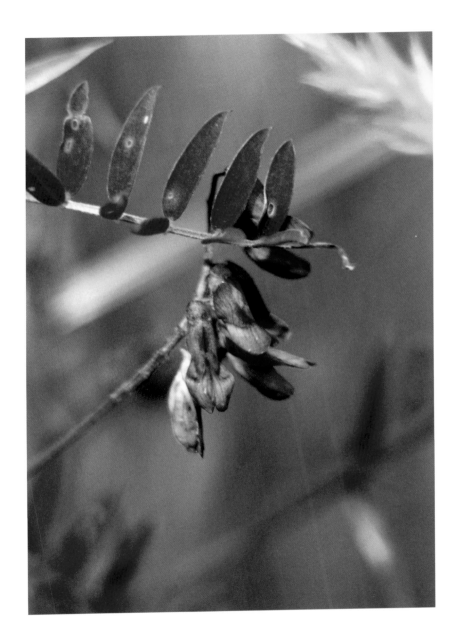

Vetch

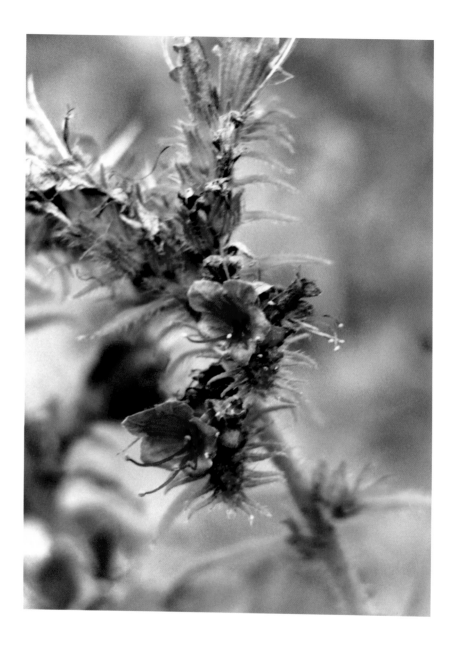

Viper's Bugloss

Viper's Bugloss
Gwiberlys, Tafod y Bwch
Echium vulgare

Description

Viper's bugloss is a medium to tall perennial. The stems and leaves are roughly hairy, and feel prickly to the touch. The leaves are lanceolate with no prominent side veins, the upper being unstalked. The flowers measure 15-20mm across and are pink turning to a vivid blue. They grow in a branched spike, with the stamens protruding from the centre of the bell-like flowers which are in bloom from May to September. The flowers are semi hidden by the sepal teeth which gives the plant a mossy appearance.

Habitat

Viper's bugloss likes growing in dry bare and waste places, and is often found on bare hillsides, sand dunes and even on shingle by the sea.

Naming History

The name bugloss stems from two Greek words; one is *bous* which means 'an ox', and the other is *glossa* meaning 'a tongue'. This is due to the shape and texture of the leaves which feel rough and similar to the surface of an ox's tongue.

The generic name *Echium* is thought to have originally derived from the Roman physician and writer Dioscorides who lived about AD 40. He knew it as *echis*, which means a 'viper' or 'snake'. He recommended it both as a cure and prevention against snake-bite, maybe because of the seed's imagined resemblance to a serpent's head. According to a poem about venomous animals written by the Greek poet and physician Nicander, this medicinal property was discovered by Alcibiades who was bitten by a snake while he slept. Presumably he was cured of his affliction with viper's bugloss. In addition the stalks of viper's bugloss are speckled resembling a snake's skin, which adds to this plant's anti-venomous characteristics.

Other uses including medicinal

Nicholas Culpeper categorised viper's bugloss as a herb of the sun. He said that the seed drunk in a little wine increased the flow of milk in nursing mothers, and the distilled water from the flowering herb could be used inwardly or outwardly to ease pains in the back, loins and kidneys.

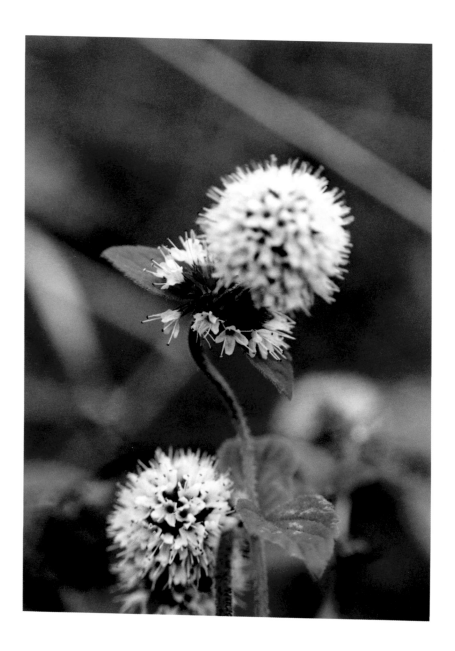

Water Mint

Water Mint
Mintys y Dŵr
Mentha aquatica

Description

This pleasantly aromatic perennial has pointed oval leaves that are toothed around the edges. The flowers which appear in July and bloom through to September are lilac or pinkish-lilac in colour, with each floret protruding from the centre of a hairy sepal tube. They grow in round heads at the top of the stems and from small branches, forming clusters around the stem.

Habitat

Water mint is both an attractive and aromatic plant, which can be found growing beside streams and in wetlands. Its flowers appear during the late summer months of July to September.

Naming History

Some people call it horse mint and Turner mentioned it in his *The Names of Herbes*, which he wrote in 1548. "Step on this Water Mint as you walk through fens or over wet meadows, and up comes the delicious damp fragrance, different from the smell of Garden Mint and not quite that of Peppermint."

Apparently Minstead in Hampshire and Minety in Wiltshire, are both towns on a tributary of the Upper Thames. They are both named after water mint, which can be translated from the Old English ('minte+sted', 'mint place', and 'minte+ea', 'mint stream').

Other uses including medicinal

According to Gerard, in the fourteenth and fifteenth centuries people would strew water mint in their chambers and places of recreation and in the dining rooms where feasts and banquets were held, presumably to give a pleasant fragrance and help to overcome other more unpleasant smells.

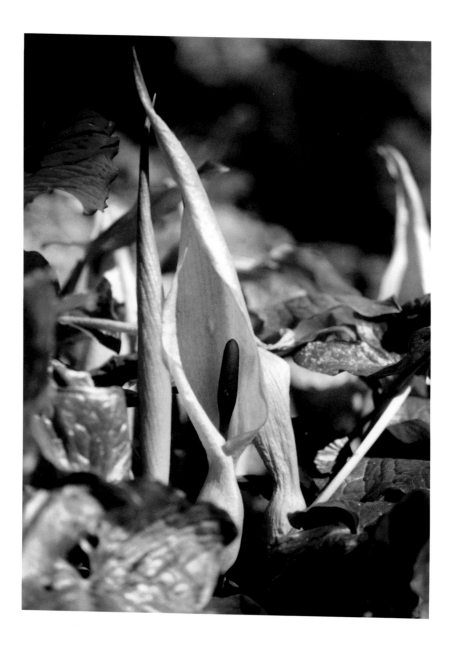

Wild Arum, Lords and Ladies, Cuckoo-Pint

Wild Arum, Lords and Ladies, Cuckoo-Pint
Pidyn y Gôg
Arum maculatum

Description

A spring search of hedgerows and woods, particularly in damp and shady areas, will often produce clumps of long, arrow-shaped leaves, dark green and mottled. In among these leaves, closer inspection will show one of the strangest flowers in the countryside. It is not brightly coloured, it does not have a pleasant smell (unless you happen to be a fly in search of carrion) and it is not a conventional shape. This is the wild arum, sometimes called cuckoo-pint or lords-and-ladies. The flower spike is in the shape of a paler green spathe or sheath, which is approximately 15-25cm in length, tapering at the top to conceal the spadix or spike. This is club-shaped and can be either yellow or have a purplish tinge. The flowers are tiny, male above female, in dense whorls capped by the conspicuous purple finger-like spadix. When they have been pollinated by a fly, they will ripen and become a cluster of bright red poisonous berries later in the season.

Habitat

Wild arum can be found growing in woods, thickets and hedgerows throughout most of Europe and the British Isles, but it is less common in more northerly regions. In the autumn, its distinctive scarlet berries are very conspicuous after the other vegetation has died back.

Naming History

The flower consists of an erect spike, the spadix, surrounded by a looser sheath, the spathe. In the minds of country folk of earlier times, it was suggestive of copulation, and for this reason was often excluded from the somewhat straitlaced Victorian flower guides.

More prosaically, the name 'cuckoo-pint' comes from the Anglo-Saxon. 'Pint' is from 'pintle' meaning a vertical projecting pin, a word still surviving today. In nautical parlance, a pintle is part of the hinge of a boat's rudder. The prefix 'cuckoo' simply means that it flowers when the cuckoo is calling. The alternative name 'arum' is from the Greek and indicates that the plant is poisonous, a reference to the fact that the flower spike eventually gives rise to a cluster of bright red and orange berries which are very poisonous. This does not, of course, apply to the starchy food called 'salep' made from the roots, which in addition to its more inter-esting properties (see below), was used by the Elizabethans for starching ruffs and other finery. For this reason, the plant was at one time also known as starchwort.

Folklore

Given the structure, the name lords-and-ladies is self-explanatory. In addition to the several connotations of the flower, and compounding the offence in Victorian eyes, the tuberous roots were the source of salep. This name derived from the Arabic source meaning 'fox's testicles', and the salep itself was popularly thought to have the effect of improving the libido, a matter of great interest to both sexes in days when few other entertainments were available.

If a young man was attending a dance, it might happen that he would place a piece of the plant in his shoe and recite the following rhyme:

> I place you in my shoe
> Let all the young girls be drawn to you.

Hopefully he would then make instant and thrilling social progress during the evening.

Not every story about this plant has sexual connotations. Apparently the Greek writer Aristotle said that when bears emerged from their long hibernation, they used the properties of this plant to soothe their sore paws which they had chewed upon through the long winter to relieve their hunger. Equally the mottled leaves show that traditionally this was one of the plants that grew at the foot of the cross, and was spotted by some of Christ's blood.

Other uses including medicinal

The wild arum is a surprisingly versatile plant. Juice expressed from the root has cleansing properties and has been used as a soap substitute, especially in Switzerland. It must have been effective because in some parts it was said to remove freckles, which seems slightly drastic. The dried root was also powdered and known as 'Cyprus Powder' (poudre de Chypre), not to be confused with the perfume Chypre which was made from Sandalwood, and was popular at one time in Paris as a cosmetic face powder. Should you suffer from gout, a hot poultice of wild arum berries and ox dung is said to bring relief to the affected limb, though possibly not to your social engagements.

Wild Daffodil
Lili Bengam, Cenhinen Pedr
Narcissus pseudonarcissus

Description

These beautiful yellow flowers are a welcome sight in early spring, after the long bleak months of winter. Sometimes called 'jonquil' from the Spanish *jonquillo* meaning 'rush', owing to the rush-like appearance of the leaves, it is exciting to see their green shoots coming up through the dark earth.

The wild daffodil is smaller than the cultivated variety. The flowers are pale yellow, five-petalled with a darker central trumpet. They appear during the early spring months of March to April, although following a mild winter, they may be seen flowering as early as January or February. They are solitary on a leafless stem, growing from the clump of spear-like leaves, which appear above ground before the flowers. The daffodil is the national emblem of Wales, and a bloom is proudly worn on 1st March, St David's Day.

Habitat

One of the loveliest sights in early spring, is a carpet of wild daffodils covering the woodland floor. Daffodils are now frequently planted along roadsides and motorways, and it may be difficult to tell the cultivated varieties from the generally smaller and more delicate wild type.

Naming History

The generic name *Narcissus* comes from Greek mythology. Narcissus was a very vain young man who was obsessed with his own reflection. He would spend many hours just admiring his face in the water, until he fell in love with his own reflection and rejected the advances of Echo. She was a mountain nymph, the servant of the goddess Hera, and through her unrequited love for Narcissus pined away day by day until only her voice was left. She haunted the mountains and spent her time in mimicking every voice or sound she heard. Narcissus was punished by Hera for his callous treatment of her servant Echo by being changed into the flower which now bears his name.

Another name for daffodils is 'Lent lilies' because they are in flower during Lent and in time for decorating the churches for Easter. When they saw the first daffodil of spring, country children would recite:

Daff-a-down-dilly has come to town
In a yellow petticoat and a green gown.

Some folk used to believe that it was unlucky to pick daffodils and bring them into the house especially when the hens are sitting on eggs, because this could cause fewer chicks to hatch. Others thought it was because of the way they hang their heads. It was also considered extremely unlucky if the first spring daffodil you saw had its head drooping towards the ground instead of upright. In fact in mediaeval times a drooping daffodil was thought to be an omen of death. However, in Wales it was believed that the person who found the first daffodil of spring would have more gold than silver for the forthcoming year, although pointing at a daffodil would prevent it from blooming.

The Victorians were particularly fond of picking wild daffodils and ran 'Daffodil Specials' to the west country on the Great Western Railway. Indeed, as late as the 1930s a 'Daffodil Special' line ran between Gloucester and the Royal Forest of Dean. Children used to sell the daffodils, though not for money as it was considered bad luck to sell daffodils for cash. They were exchanged for pins instead, hence a possible origin of the phrase 'pin money'.

Other uses including medicinal

Daffodils were used in medicine but mainly externally. According to Culpeper all the white daffodils were governed by Venus, and the yellow came under Mars. The bruised roots were boiled with dried barley-meal and used to heal wounds, and mixed with honey it was also applied to sprains and aching joints. This herb is not recommended for modern use, although a homeopathic medicine is made from the bulb and used particularly for treating bronchitis and whooping cough.

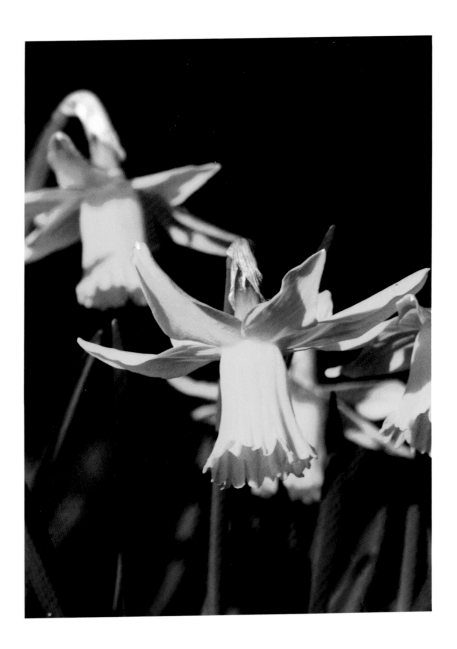

Wild Daffodil

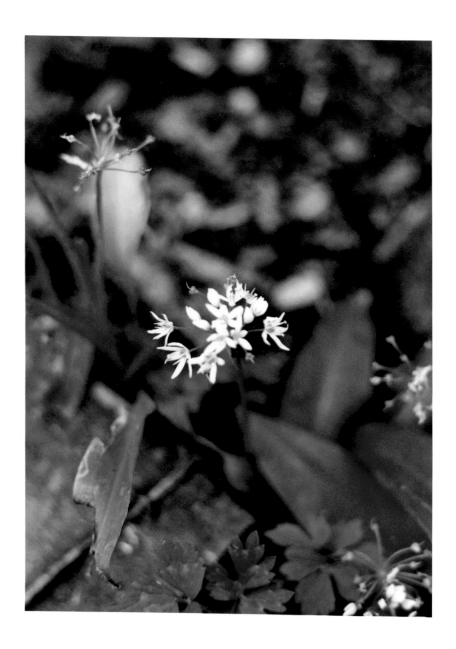

Wild Garlic or Ramsons

Wild Garlic or Ramsons
Craf y Geifr
Allium ursinum

Description

It is obvious by its name that this attractive plant has a strong garlic smell. In fact anywhere this plant is found growing there is often a strong smell of garlic in the air. The white star-like flowers appear during the months of April to June forming an 'umbel' around the head of the triangular-shaped stem. The broad elliptical leaves grow directly from the roots. They are bright green and smell of garlic.

Habitat

Wild garlic is a plant that likes shade. It can be found growing in carpets on woodland floors and on shady banks.

Naming History

The common name 'ramsons' comes from the Anglo-Saxon word *hramsa*, meaning 'rank', which perfectly describes the strong smell and taste of the plant. Milk and butter can both be tainted if wild garlic is eaten by dairy cows. The generic name *Allium* is the classical Latin name for garlic, although its original meaning is obscure. The specific name *ursinum* means, surprisingly enough, 'pertaining to bears'. This is either from an old belief that bears were fond of the strong taste of garlic, or that garlic was considered to be strong and coarse, like a bear.

The Old English name for ramsons was *bramsa*, evolving to 'hramson', and eventually to ramson. There are towns in England which take their names from ramsons. Evidently the plant grew there and probably still does. These include Ramsbottom in Lancashire, meaning 'Ramson Valley', and Ramsey in Essex and again in Huntingdonshire, meaning 'Ramson Island'. Some other attractive country names include; 'brandy bottles' from Wiltshire, 'onion flower' from Somerset and 'Devil's posy' from Dorset, presumably because of the plant being used against evil spirits.

Folklore

Garlic placed on mole hills was said to draw moles from the ground, and it was universally used in cock fighting because the 'heady' smell was thought to stimulate the birds to fight. In addition to this a concoction was made which included garlic. It was called 'vinegar of the four thieves' and was said to protect its users from infection. Surprisingly enough it was also used by robbers of plague victims, possibly because garlic is said to keep away evil spirits. It was also believed that it helped to cure measles. A piece of home-spun linen was torn into nine pieces and then powdered garlic from nine bulbs was then spread onto each piece. These pieces were then wrapped around the child, who was then nursed for nine days, after which the linen was then buried in the garden and hopefully the child would recover. What is the significance of number nine I do not know, beyond the fact that it is a 'mystic number' which often occurred in pagan worship.

Garlic was used as a popular remedy in south Wales. In the village of Llanfallteg in Carmarthen, evidence has been found that people placed garlic in their socks before retiring to bed, as a remedy for a common head cold. They believed that the strong aroma would work its way to the head by the morning.

Garlic was also considered a remedy for snake bites in humans as well as in animals, because it was believed that garlic travelled through the bloodstream quicker than the venom.

Other uses including medicinal

John Gerard quoted an old English recipe which stated that a sauce was made from the leaves of wild garlic and butter, which was delicious poured over fish.

Wild Pansy
Llysieuyn y Drindod, Pansi
Viola tricolor

Description

The pansy is a familiar sight in flowerbeds and hanging baskets, but the less famil-iar wild version is just as attractive. The typically yellow and/or violet flowers are up to 25mm across, carried on low stems among the broad oval leaves. The flow-ering period is from April to November. Pansies grow in bare and grassy places and sand dunes, tolerating sun and shade.

Naming History

In the sixteenth century the name 'heartsease' was applied to both pansies and wallflowers. In 1548 William Turner likened the wild pansy to "two faces in a hood", because it gave the impression that the two side petals were kissing inside the hood made by the upper and lower petals. He said it looked as if the kiss eased the heart, hence the name 'Heartsease', but it was also called 'three-faces-in-one-hood' or 'under one hood', because the large lower petal represented the girl, and the petals on either side of her, her lovers, of whom one was left out, giving rise to the further names of 'love in idleness' and 'love in vain.' In his play *A Midsummer Night's Dream*, Shakespeare made Oberon squeeze the juice of 'love-in-idleness' into Titania's eyes, which made her fall in love with the ass-headed Bottom, when she awoke. However this pretty flower was considered to be asso-ciated too much with wantonness, so it was Christianised and called *'Trinitatis herba'*, 'The herb of the blessed Trinity' on account of its three colours in unity.

Another rather rueful name is 'stepmothers', this is because of the large richly coloured lower petal, representing the stepmother, the two side petals which signify her own children, and the two upper, half-hidden petals the neglected step-children. Other country names include; 'butterfly flower', 'kiss me quick' and 'kiss behind the garden gate'.

Folklore

Superstitions have a tendency to dwell on bad luck or unfortunate choices, so it is perhaps not surprising to find many relating to death. In the case of pansies, it was thought picking a flower with dew or rain on it would cause the death of a loved one, so was naturally avoided. But picking a pansy on a fine day would cause it to rain, possibly a valuable attribute in dry countries.

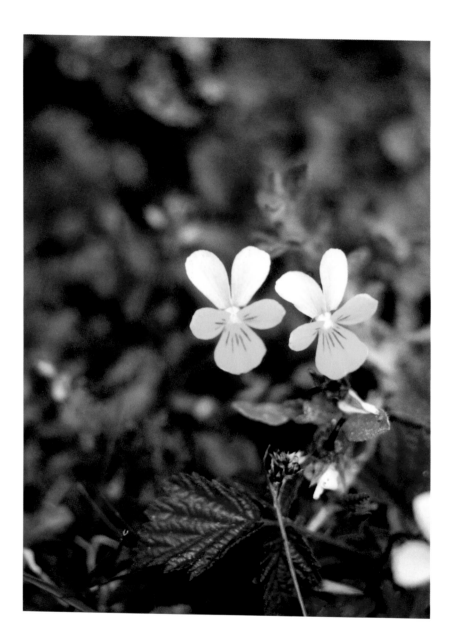

Wild Pansy

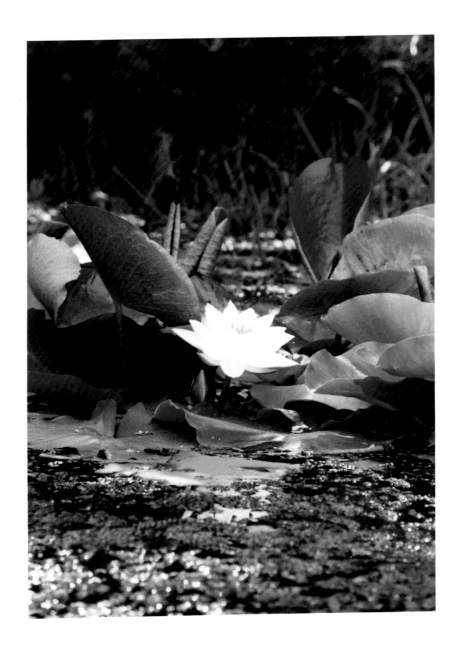

White Water Lily

White Water Lily
Lili'r Dŵr
Nymphaea alba L.

Description

As the name suggests, these plants are aquatic. Rooted in the mud at the bottom of a pond, a cluster of stems arises and is supported by large flat leaves that float on the surface. From June to September, additional stems produce large, multi-petalled white flowers, up to 200mm across. Although it is not easy to sample it, the flowers do have a pleasant scent. Water lilies are descended from one of the first families of plants to produce true flowers. These flowers are fertilized by beetles, and most blooms provide little payment to their visitors other than the pollen itself.

Habitat

Water lilies grow in still, shallow water with a thick layer of mud or silt on the bottom. If it is too deep (more than 600-900mm) then stems cannot reach the surface.

Naming History

According to William Turner's *The Grete Herball* of 1526, Elizabethan apothecaries called both species by the name of *nenuphar*. This is a contrived word, which came by way of mediaeval Latin from *nilotpala*, the Sanskrit for the Blue Lotus of India which is *Nymphaea stellata*.

The beauty of the water lily is well described by some of the local names which include 'lady of the lake' in Cheshire and in Donegal, Ireland, 'swan amongst the flowers'. Maybe the white flower gives the impression of a lady's dress floating on the surface of the water.

Folklore

Carvings of the yellow water lily dating from the thirteenth century can be found in certain churches, including Westminster Abbey and Bristol Cathedral. It was obviously a favourite of the sculptor who worked on the Angel Choir at Lincoln, since the example there shows an artistic waviness of the leaves.

Another name for the yellow water lily is 'brandy bottle' or 'can-dock' in the Highlands of Scotland, because the flowers smell of the stale dregs of brandy, or the dregs of a sweet white wine. When the sepals and petals have been removed, the capsule represents a green-glazed wine carafe. Therefore the word 'can-dock' means a plant which has leaves like a dock and capsules like carafes.

Other uses including medicinal

The yellow water lily *Nuphar lutea* is the true wild version. It is smaller than the white and has a longer stem. It is quite rare. Both the yellow and the white varieties have had some curious applications. The rhizomes of the yellow water lily were soaked in tar and applied to the head to prevent baldness (personally I would have thought this would have induced it), whereas the black rhizomes of the white water lily were steeped in red wine and given for the treatment of leucorrhoea. Over-sexed Elizabethans ate the seeds and sprinkled the powdered rhizomes over meat, or drank them in broth to cool themselves down.

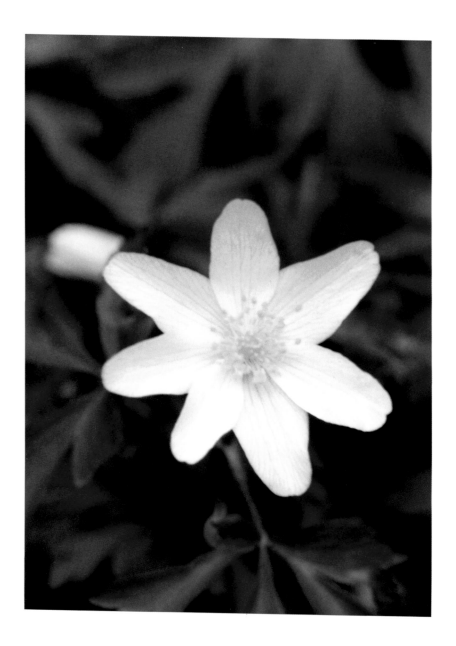

Wood Anemone

Wood Anemone
Blodyn y Gwynt
Anemone nemorosa

Description

The characteristic deeply-cut leaves of the wood anemone appear in the spring shortly before the flowers. The solitary white flowers are usually about 20-40mm across, with six to eight petals, sometimes tinged with pink on the underside, and a cluster of yellow anthers in the centre. The flowers open during the daylight hours and close at night and during dull weather.

Habitat

Wood anemones flower in open woodland during the spring months of March, April and May, before the woodland canopy comes into leaf and shades the woodland floor. They like rich soils and plenty of sunlight and are mostly found flowering in deciduous woods such as sycamore woods and coppices. They make a wonderful sight in spring, with their carpets of white after the long dreary winter months.

Naming History

All species of anemones are referred to as wind flowers. According to the Roman naturalist Pliny, the flowers will not open until the wind blows, but it is rather more likely that it is because they nod and shake their heads in the wind. When the sun moves across the sky to set in the west, the windflowers move their heads round to follow it and thereby make the most of the sunlight.

The original Anemone was a beautiful nymph from Greek mythology. Zephyr, the god of the west wind, fell helplessly in love with her. Unfortunately Zephyr was already married and his wife Flora was, perhaps not surprisingly, jealous. She maliciously turned Anemone into a small flower. Thereafter Zephyr deserted her and went back to his wife and doubtful domestic harmony, but Boreas, god of the north wind, saw his opportunity and wooed her in the spring hoping she would open to his chillier charms.

The origin of the anemone, however, goes back further in time than the Greeks. There is early evidence of cultivated anemones blooming in Egypt (around 1570-1085 BC), although the species is unknown. The anemone features in early Egyptian artwork along with the cornflower, poppy and chrysanthemum.

Folklore

Culpeper associated anemones with the planet Venus, but it has been considered by some as a fairy plant because the elves were said to have painted the red veins on the petals. Anemones act as natural barometers, and will start to close their petals in a tent-like fashion at the approach of night or at the onset of a sudden shower. Country folk believed this was done by fairies who lived inside the petals and pulled the 'curtains' around them.

In some regions it was believed that picking a wood anemone would induce a thunderstorm, which gave it the country name of 'thunderbolt' and meant that it would certainly not be a flower to put in one's buttonhole. Because of their unpleasant smell they are also sometimes called 'smell foxes', so you wouldn't want to wear it in your buttonhole anyway! Although they are fragile in appearance, wood anemones are in fact strong and well able to withstand the wind; but they do not last long in water and wither quickly if picked.

Other uses including medicinal

During the seventeenth century when Nicholas Culpeper was practising his herbal medicine, the wood anemone was considered a very useful plant. The leaves were boiled and the body was then bathed with the decoction as a cure for leprosy. The juice was extracted by stamping on the leaves and was then sniffed up the nose to "purge the head mightily". The root when chewed was an expectorant and "procureth much spitting and bringeth away watery and phlegmatic humours" and was therefore excellent for relieving lethargy.

The roots could also be made into an ointment to anoint the eyelids and give relief to inflammations of the eyes. The same ointment was considered excellent for cleansing malignant and corroding ulcers.

Nowadays it is made into a tincture and used to treat nervous headaches and asthma. It is also sometimes used to help combat the symptoms of arthritis and rheumatism.

Wood Sorrel
Suran y Coed
Oxalis acetosella

Description

If you are walking through deciduous woodland in late spring, your eye may be caught by a patch of shamrock-like leaves, paler green than most, and growing in small clusters close to the ground. This is wood sorrel and, despite its name, it is no relation to common sorrel. Wood sorrel is a very interesting plant because it produces two forms of flower. The first is the familiar white, five-petalled, lilac-veined bell-shaped flower, that we see on the woodland floor. These flowers close their petals in cloudy weather, or towards the evening, and they wilt quickly in strong sunlight. This flower however, produces very little seed and is only there to attract insects for pollination. The second form of flowers bloom prolifically in the summer near the ground on short stems, and seldom open, but these are the flowers that make most of the seeds to continue the next generation.

Habitat

Wood sorrel, as the name implies, is a woodland plant. More particularly it grows in shady places on the woodland floor. The bright green three-lobed leaves may be seen at any time from early spring through to autumn, often in association with mossy clumps or wood anemones, but the spring flowers appear before the tree canopy is established and disappear as the shade increases. The summer flowers are shade tolerant. In general wood sorrel prefers an acid soil.

Naming History

The common name 'sorrel' is said to have come from the French name *surelle* which originally came from the German word *suur* which means 'sour'. The leaves of this plant have a slightly sour, lemony taste, which some people find pleasant in salads. Wood sorrel also likes growing on acid soil, this may help to explain the scientific name *oxalis* which comes from the Greek *oxys*, which means 'acid', but it is most likely due to the strong taste of the leaves.

Folklore

The three-lobed leaves look very like the familiar Irish shamrock and together with the rather similar clover were once said to be the shamrock used by St

Patrick to illustrate the Holy Trinity to a rural audience. This leads into an attractive story about a fifth century monk who visited Ireland to teach the gospel and try to convert the pagans to Christianity. He had a hard time convincing them, and was mocked and jeered at in every way. He had difficulty in explaining to them about the Holy Trinity, and finally resorted to using a wood sorrel leaf to demonstrate to them that "if it's possible for three leaves to grow on one stem, then it is possible for three people to be one". A tradition says that this circumstance prompted the Irish to adopt Saint Patrick as their patron saint.

Another ecclesiastical connection is the mediaeval name of 'alleluia', deriving from the appearance of the leaves around Easter when 'alleluia is song agayn'. Evidence of this plant's appeal can be found in a number of old churches where its trefoil shape can sometimes be found among the roof carving motifs.

Other names for wood sorrel are 'cuckowes meat' and 'wood sour', because this plant was thought to benefit the cuckoo. Some of the old apothecaries thought that it was the food of the cuckoo, and the cuckoo's song could be heard most when the plant was flowering.

Other uses including medicinal

Wood sorrel was considered sacred by the Celts, and the druids had a profound respect for its magical properties. In later years the mediaeval herbalists referred to it as highly therapeutic in the treatment of fevers and reducing bodily inflammations. So much so in fact that the Elizabethan herbalist John Gerard was prompted to say "When stamped and used for greene sauce, it is good for them that have sicke and feeble stomackes, for it strengtheneth the stomacke and procureth appetite". In fact a tincture made from the roots was thought to be good for treating problems involving the liver, bladder and kidneys. A useful wound herb, a tincture of the leaves could be used to wash the mouth of a wound, and it was considered excellent for reducing the swelling and pain in sprains.

Also due to the shape of the leaves, "broad at the ends, cut in the middle and sharp towards the stalk", it was thought that wood sorrel would be beneficial in the treatment of heart disease.

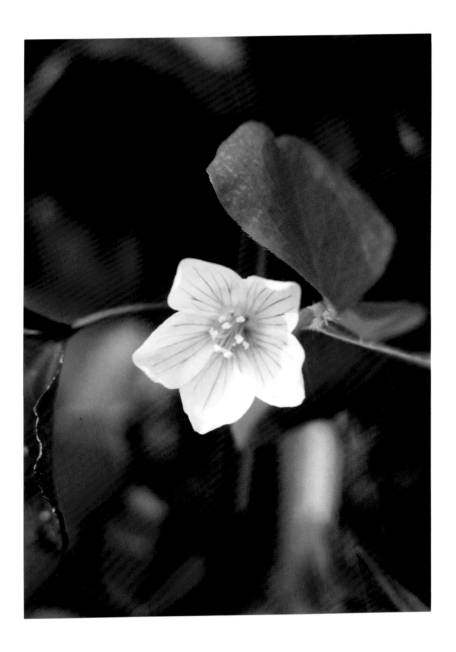

Wood Sorrel

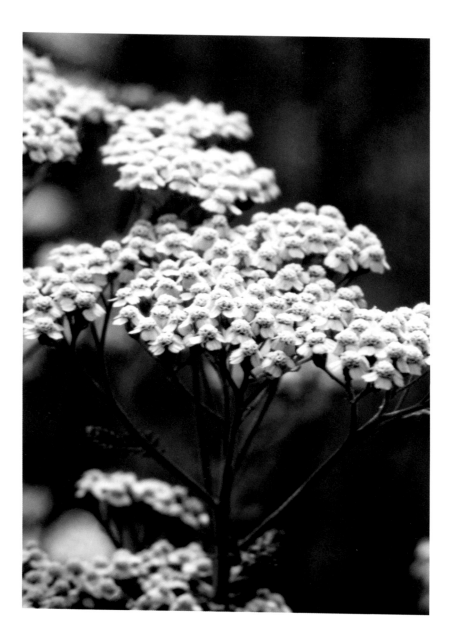

Yarrow

Yarrow
Milddail, Llysiau Gwaedlif
Achillea millefolium

Description

Yarrow is a common perennial which grows up to 50cm (20in) tall. Its flowers, which appear from June to November, can be either pale pink or white and grow in flat, umbel-like clusters. Its leaves grow as dark green feathery fronds, which gives yarrow its other name of 'milfoil' or 'thousand leaf'.

Habitat

Yarrow can be found growing in open grassy places, such as meadows, waste ground and wayside verges. It is not a tall plant so it does not grow in areas of long grass. It is very common, and grows across temperate Europe and in parts of North America.

Naming History

Yarrow is a native European plant, with a long history as a wound healer. In fact one of the Welsh names for this plant is 'Llysiau gwaedlif', because of its property for resisting blood flow. In classical times it was called *herba militaris*, because it was used to staunch war wounds. This is portrayed by the generic name *Achillea*, after the Greek hero Achilles. In the first century the Greek physician Dioscorides describes how Achilles discovered the herb Yarrow and found it beneficial in curing the wounds caused by iron weapons.

A more sinister side of yarrow is shown by its other names of 'mother-die', or 'fever plant'. Apparently it was considered unlucky to bring into the house because it was thought to cause sickness.

Folklore

Yarrow was a popular plant used by maids for divination. If a maid lived in Sussex, she had to pick a sprig from the grave of a young man, or at the time of the full moon if she resided in the West Country, whereas in Herefordshire she would have to pick it from a churchyard that she had never visited before. She would then take the sprig of yarrow back to her house, wrap it in flannel and, before going to bed, place it under her pillow, while at the same time reciting the following verse:

Thou pretty herb of Venus tree,
Thy true name is Yarrow
Now who my bosom friend must be
Pray tell thou me tomorrow.

Hopefully the next morning when she cut through the yarrow's stem, she would see her future husband's initials inside. The Suffolk maidens appeared to be more desperate. This rhyme appeared in the *Folk Lore Record* of 1878:

Green arrow, green arrow, you wears a white bow;
If my love love me, my nose will bleed now;
If my love don't love me, it'ont bleed a drop;
If my love do love me, twill bleed every drop.

Despite the Suffolk maidens, yarrow used to be called 'nose-bleed', because it was believed that a headache or migraine could be relieved by pushing yarrow leaves up the nostrils and thus inducing a nose bleed. This was thought to ease the pressure and therefore ease the pain, of the headache at any rate.

In County Donegal on the eve of the 30th April, youths and maids would cut a square sod of earth which contained, amongst other things, yarrow. They would place this under their pillow and, if they remained silent between the times of cutting the sod and falling asleep they would hopefully dream of their future sweetheart. This custom was thought to have been introduced by Scottish settlers.

Another Irish custom from Belfast states that on the eve of the first of May a girl would pick nine leaves of yarrow and quote:

Yarrow for yarrow, if yarrow you be
By this time tomorrow
My true love to see.
The colour of his hair
The clothes he does wear
The first words he will speak
When he comes to court me.

She should then place the leaves under her pillow, and hopefully she would dream of her future spouse.

Country people used to have a great fear of the supernatural. They used to wear a sprig of yarrow on their persons, or tie it onto a cradle to protect themselves from witches. If a bunch of yarrow was hung up in the house on St John's Eve, it was thought to keep sickness away from the family for at least a year. It was also used rather like a 'good luck' charm at a wedding. If some was eaten during a wedding feast, it was meant to ensure that the couple would love each other and stay together for a least seven years. In the Hebridean Islands off the coast of northern Scotland, it was believed that if a leaf of yarrow was held against the eyes, it would give that person second sight.

Other uses including medicinal

For a long time yarrow has been taken as a strengthening, bitter-tasting tonic and all kinds of bitter drinks have been made from it. Tea made from hay or yarrow was thought to be beneficial to sheep, and yarrow tea was (and perhaps still is) drunk by people to cure migraines and to treat cystitis. It was also thought to be beneficial for bladder weakness and for reducing a fever, and for easing a sore throat. To improve blood circulation, the Welsh would use the following method to make (yet another) tea:

1) Collect the top shoots of the plant and hang to dry naturally
2) Boil some of the crushed plant in 1 pint of water
3) Add a spoonful of sugar if desired
4) Take three times a day

It is said that chewing the leaves reduces the pain in toothache, and it is good for strengthening the stomach, back and kidneys.

The druids used the stalk to predict the weather during the different seasons, but I have not been able to find out any further information about this.

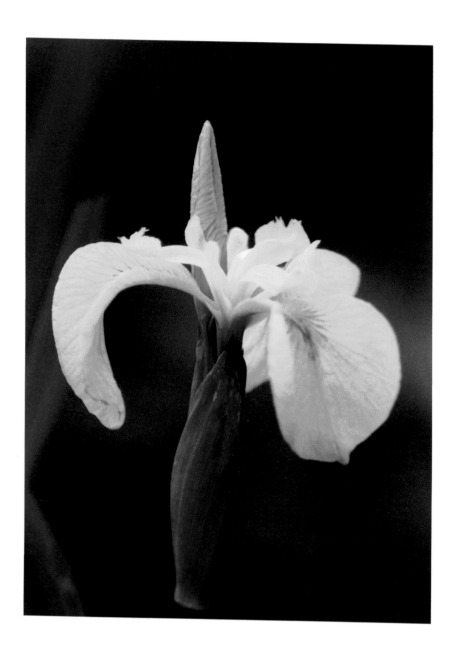

Yellow Flag Iris

Yellow Flag Iris
Gellhesg
Iris pseudacorus

Description

This is the commonest of the wild irises and is distinguished from the others by its longer and narrower leaves. It is a very tall plant, sometimes growing to more than 2.1metres. It grows in large clumps, spreading by means of its thick rhizomes. The sword-shaped leaves are long, thick and narrow and rise directly from the often conspicuous rhizomes.

The large splendid flowers which appear during the summer months of June to August, have three spreading and sometimes bearded petals (falls) and three erect and twisted ones which comprise the centre (standards). The petals all narrow towards the base, and the three large stigmas are petal-like in their appearance.

Habitat

Yellow flag irises are always found growing in large clumps by fresh water, especially by rivers, streamsides and in marshes.

Naming History

These spectacular waterside flowers are not a native British plant, but were introduced into mediaeval Britain in the ninth century. The common name 'yellow flag' refers to the colour of the flower and the way the petals hang loosely from the flowering spike, from the old verb 'to flag' meaning to droop or to hang. It may also have something to do with the mediaeval word 'flakken' meaning to flap. In fact Louis VII (1137-1180) was so fond of these flowers that they were spread thickly on the French flag in the twelfth century, but the number was reduced to three in honour of the Holy Trinity by Charles V two hundred years later.

The generic name *iris* is a Latin word for 'rainbow' because of the many and varied colours of this family of plants. Iris was the Greek goddess of the rainbow, or the rainbow itself. In classical mythology she was the messenger of the gods, and of Juno in particular, and the rainbow is the bridge or road let down from heaven for her accommodation.

Other uses including medicinal

The yellow flag iris had many uses both practically and for play. Children used its thick wide leaves to make boats, and sent them floating down the streams. The rhizomes were used to produce a black ink and a dark green dye, and it has been maintained that the seeds can be ground down and roasted and made into a very passable coffee. The seeds also produce an oil which has a very sweet aroma. This used to be used in mediaeval and Elizabethan homes to keep the air fresh and free from nasty odours. In some places yellow flag would be strewn in the church in front of the bride and groom, to be crushed underfoot and release the lovely scent as the couple walked down the aisle.

Yellow Rattle
Clychau'r Meirch, Pen Siarad, Pwrs Broga
Rhinanthus minor

Description

Yellow rattle is a member of the figwort family, the rather unattractively named *Scrophulariaceae*, as can be seen from the two-lipped flowers, but does not seem, at first sight, to have any other distinguishing features. Surprisingly enough this family also contains the foxglove. If, however, you are patient and wait a month or two until the plant goes to seed, the origin of the 'rattle' name will become clear. The flowers give way to seed pods, the whole stem dries and stiffens further and, if touched or shaken, the loose seeds within make a distinct rattling, rustling sound. If you pick the seedhead and shake it, the seeds will be shaken out of the pods, and the plant has successfully dispersed them. This is not to say, of course, that the seed-head has been designed by evolution to be picked and shaken for a moment's diversion by casual walkers, but the wind sweeping over the grass or animals brushing through the field will do the job just as effectively.

Habitat

Throughout the summer in grassy meadows, the attractive upright flowerheads of yellow rattle can be seen, usually in patches among the other plants. It is a semi-parasite on grasses, the roots sucking nutriment from the grass roots and ultimately killing the grass and resulting in fields of yellow rattle. On account of this capability, it is regarded with disfavour by farmers who maintain grazing pasture.

Naming History

The generic name *Rhinanthus*, in translation from the Greek, means 'snout flower', apparently on account of the fanciful resemblance to a rhinoceros head, although this may be difficult to recognise.

Folklore

In areas of Buckinghamshire the local name for yellow rattle is 'locusts' (pronounced locus), because it was supposed to have been the food of John the Baptist in the wilderness, and when the yellow rattle is in flower the hay is said to be ready for cutting.

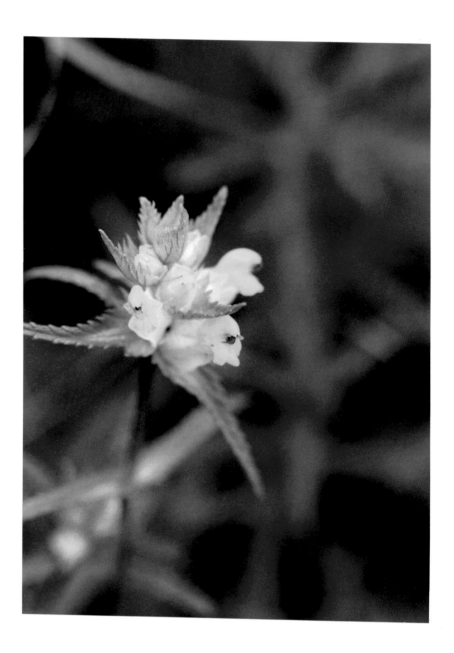

Yellow Rattle

Other uses including medicinal

Yellow rattle was considered good for coughs or dimness of the sight, especially if it was boiled with beans, and some honey. It could then be drunk or dropped directly into the eyes. Largely due to the resemblance of their medicinal properties with eyebright, red rattle and yellow rattle have both fallen from popularity as modern herbal remedies.

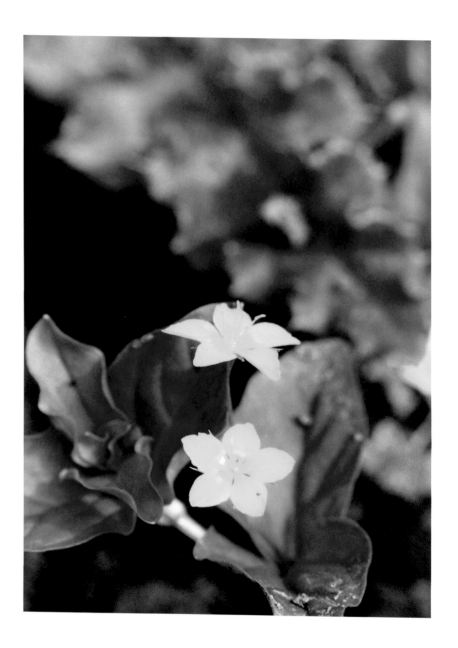

Yellow Pimpernel

Yellow Pimpernel
Gwlydd Melyn Mair, Melyn y Tywydd, Seren Felen
Lysimachia nemorum L.

Description
Not very closely related to the scarlet pimpernel, these small attractive flowers appear during the summer months of May to August. The five-petalled yellow flowers, which are hermaphrodite, are only about 12mm across and grow at intervals between the pointed oval leaves along a creeping stem. Pollination is carried out by both bees and flies.

Habitat
Yellow pimpernel favours damp and grassy places, and is often found in woodland margins.

Naming History
The common name yellow pimpernel was given to this little flower to distinguish it from the scarlet pimpernel *Anagallis arvensis*. It does have some attractive local names too, some of which are closely linked with the Virgin Mary. In Wiltshire it is known as 'Star Flower', in Ireland it is called *'seamar Mhuire'*, 'Mary's Clover', in Gaelic it is called *'lus Cholumcille'*, 'St Colum Cille's plant' and in Welsh it is given the pretty name of 'gwlydd melyn Mair', 'Mary's yellow stem'.

Other uses including medicinal
Yellow pimpernel has been used as an astringent to staunch bleeding. In addition, it seems to be immune to grazing by rabbits, and perhaps has an unpleasant taste.

The Amen! of nature is always a flower.

Oliver Wendell Holmes.

Bibliography

David Attenborough: *The Private Life of Plants* (BBC Books, 1995)

Margaret Baker: *Discovering The Folklore of Plants* (Shire Publications, 1969)

Andrew Chevallier: *Encyclopaedia of Medicinal Plants* (Dorling Kindersley, 1969)

Rev Hilderic Friend: *Flowers and Folk Lore* (Swan, Sonnenschein, Le Bas and Lowery, 1886)

Geoffrey Grigson: *The Englishman's Flora* (Phoenix House Ltd, 1958)

Robin Gwyndaf: *Welsh Folk Tales** (Welsh Folk Museum, 1970)

David Hoffmann: *Welsh Herbal Medicine* (Abercastle Publications, 1978)

Ann Jenkins: *Llysiau Rhinweddol** (Gwasg Gomer, 1982)

T Gwynn Jones: *Welsh Folklore of Wales* (London, 1930)

Mary Jones: *Llysiau Llesol** (JD Lewis, 1978)

Michael Jordan: *Plants of Mystery and Magic* (Cassell Illustrated, 1997)

JR Press, botanical consultant: *Culpeper's Colour Herbal* (W Foulsham & Co Ltd, 1983)

John E Stevens: *Discovering Wild Plant Names* (Shire Publications, 1973)

Marie Trevelyan: *Folklore and Folkstories of Wales* (EP, 1909)

Roy Vickery: *Dictionary of Plant Lore* (Oxford University Press, 1995)

Philip Wilkinson and Adam Hart-Davies: *What the Romans Did for Us* (Macmillan, 2001)

Brewer's Dictionary of Phrase and Fable (Cassell, 1970)

Chambers Biographical Dictionary (1990)

Collins English Dictionary (1979)

Shorter Oxford English Dictionary (1972)

*My special thanks go to Robin Gwyndaf of the Museum of Welsh Life for the loan of these books, and to Nicolas Walker for giving me the run of the museum library, plus personal communications too numerous to list!

Index of English names

Index of Welsh names

Index of scientific names

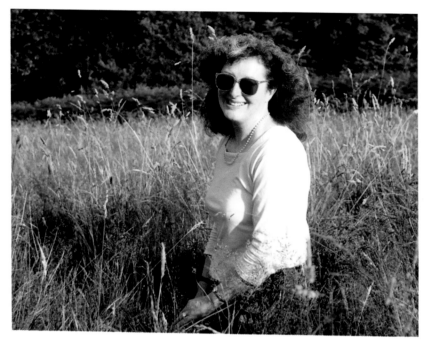

photo: Sarah Lawton

Jocelyne Lawton

Jocelyne Lawton is a 'laboratory technician turned naturalist' and an enthusiastic self-taught photographer. She is married to a countryside warden and lives in the Bryngarw Country Park near Bridgend, where many of the photographs in this book were taken. She has two cats, Benedic and Beatrice, who often accompany her on her photographic trips.

Flowers and Fables is her first book.